AIDS EDUCATION

AIDS EDUCATION

Reaching Diverse Populations

Edited by Melinda K. Moore
and Martin L. Forst

PRAEGER

Westport, Connecticut
London

Library of Congress Cataloging-in-Publication Data

AIDS education : reaching diverse populations / edited by Melinda K.
  Moore, Martin L. Forst.
       p.   cm.
    Includes bibliographical references and index.
    ISBN 0–275–94904–4 (alk. paper)
    1. AIDS (Disease)—United States—Prevention—Cross-cultural
  studies.   2. Community health services—United States.   I. Moore,
  Melinda.   II. Forst, Martin Lyle.
  RA644.A25A3593   1996
  362.1'969792'00973—dc20   95–49715

British Library Cataloguing in Publication Data is available.

Library of Congress Catalog Card Number: 95–49715
ISBN: 0–275–94904–4

First published in 1996

Praeger Publishers, 88 Post Road West, Westport, CT 06881
An imprint of Greenwood Publishing Group, Inc.

Printed in the United States of America

The paper used in this book complies with the
Permanent Paper Standard issued by the National
Information Standards Organization (Z39.48–1984).

10 9 8 7 6 5 4 3 2

][—————————————————

Contents

][———————

Tables and Figures

FIGURES

TABLES

AIDS EDUCATION

1

Introduction: Targeting AIDS Education and Prevention Programs

Melinda K. Moore
and Martin L. Forst

Since physicians Linda Laubenstein and Kenneth Hymes first reported the occurrence of a rare cancer—Kaposi's sarcoma—affecting gay men in New York City in 1979 and the subsequent identification of human immunodeficiency virus (HIV) in 1984, HIV infection has continued to spread rapidly in the United States and throughout the world. World Health Organization epidemiologists calculate that as of 1993 approximately eight to ten million people were infected worldwide and estimate that by the year 2000, more than forty million people will be infected with HIV and five to six million will have been diagnosed with acquired immune deficiency syndrome (AIDS).

As of June 1995, 476,899 AIDS cases had been reported in the United States to the Centers for Disease Control and Prevention. A total of 291,815 AIDS-related deaths had been reported in the same period, representing a 61.1 percent mortality rate. Nationally, by the end of 1994, gay/bisexual men constituted 52.0 percent of known adult AIDS cases, injection drug users (IDUs) 32.0 percent, heterosexuals 7.0 percent, hemophiliac/transfusion recipients 2.5 percent, infants and children 1.0 percent, and adult "undetermined" 8.0 percent. Total deaths from AIDS increased from 131 in 1981 to 294,473 by the end of 1994. This represents more than a 2,200-fold increase in just fourteen years.

HIV/AIDS EFFECTS IN DIFFERENT POPULATIONS

HIV/AIDS does not affect all segments of the population equally. Data from the Centers for Disease Control and Prevention reveal the greatest increases in diagnosed AIDS cases in the United States are among women, African-Americans, Latinos, persons exposed to HIV through heterosexual contact, and persons in the South. In 1994 alone, 64,300 people were newly diagnosed with AIDS. Of those, 41.2 percent were white, 39.3 percent were African-American, 18.5 percent Latino, 0.7 percent Asian, and 0.3 percent American Indian/Alaska Native.

Although the total number of AIDS cases among African-Americans and Latinos is still lower than the number of cases among whites, based on rates per 100,000 population, African-Americans and Latinos are greatly overrepresented among AIDS victims. For example, the rate for whites is 11.7 cases per 100,000, compared to 52.2 for African-Americans and 29.9 among Latinos.

In 1988, HIV/AIDS infection was the eighth leading cause of death among American women aged twenty-five to forty-four. By 1992, HIV/AIDS infection became one of the top five leading causes of death among young women. For African-American women aged fifteen to forty-four in New Jersey and New York, AIDS has been the leading cause of death since in 1987.

In California between 1991 and 1992, there was a 17.6 percent increase in the number of women diagnosed with AIDS, an 18.3 percent increase among African-Americans, 9.3 percent among Latinos, and a 66.7 percent increase in the number of American Indians diagnosed with AIDS. There was also a 19.4 percent increase among injection drug users and a 15.8 percent increase in the exposure category labeled "heterosexuals." By the end of 1995, close to 100,000 AIDS cases will have been diagnosed in California, more than triple the 32,000 cases diagnosed through 1989.

For years, AIDS activists have argued that far more people have HIV/AIDS than the statistics indicated. Finally, in January 1993, the federal Centers for Disease Control and Prevention acknowledged that the activists were correct and adopted a more inclusive definition of the disease. As a result, the number of new AIDS cases was expected to almost double in 1993, to at least 90,000. The old definition, in use for five years, did not include symptoms peculiar to women and injection drug users who tested HIV positive. The new one includes several new diseases and adds an indicator: a drop in the level of a patient's master immune cells to about one-fifth the normal level.

EDUCATION AND PREVENTION

Each year since statistics have been kept on the incidence and prevalence of HIV/AIDS in the United States, the number of those infected has grown exponentially. And, while billions of dollars have been spent on HIV/AIDS-related research, there is still no cure in sight. Moreover, researchers, initially hopeful of developing a vaccine to prevent contracting HIV or a medicine to stop the progression of the disease once contracted, are now increasingly pessimistic about the development of either in the near future.

Public-health prevention education is generally regarded to lie at the heart of any comprehensive strategy to stem the spread of HIV infection. In this regard, the news is somewhat more optimistic— the risk-reduction measures which need to be adopted are relatively few (practicing safer sex behaviors and safe needle-using practices) and are relatively inexpensive to implement. However, the simplicity of the needed changes belies the complex social, cultural, and economic issues behind these edicts.

More knowledge has been accumulated about how HIV is transmitted and how it can be prevented than is available for most of the other leading causes of deaths in the United States. Through this accumulated knowledge, we face unprecedented opportunities in the 1990s for implementing prevention programs to slow or even stop new infections. Yet there is growing pessimism among providers about effecting behavior change in all but the most motivated.

To be effective, education programs must target the specific behaviors that place people at risk for HIV infection. Toward this end, epidemiological studies have identified certain needle-using and sexual behaviors, called high-risk behaviors, that increase the probability of HIV infection and transmission. These studies have also determined the prevalence of these high-risk behaviors among some groups.

What remains more elusive, however, is an understanding of why people engage in risky behaviors. For example, a lack of understanding of what causes sexual risk-taking and the extent to which these causes are culturally based is likely to compromise the effectiveness of intervention efforts aimed at changing these behaviors and preventing the further spread of HIV/AIDS.

It is difficult to work in the midst of an epidemic that continues to go unchecked, killing thousands of relatively young people each year. The authors believe that, as a coping strategy, many health educators have convinced themselves that behavior change is easily achieved. This is not the case. Changing behaviors, particularly sexual behaviors that often have a deeply embedded cultural base, is a monumental task. Moreover, we cannot assume that all individuals have sufficient power in their relationships with husbands, lovers, and friends to effect change, even if they desired to do so.

EDUCATION EFFECTIVENESS IN DIFFERENT POPULATIONS

Education efforts have had varying levels of success within particular communities. Some people have been able to change their behaviors more easily than others. For example, while research suggests that educational interventions have been relatively successful at changing the sexual practices of gay white males, among women of color and sexual partners of injection drug users effecting behavior change has been much more difficult.

Yet even among gay white males, epidemiologists are also recounting a growing "generation gap" in AIDS awareness. Many youths in the gay community are apparently practicing high-risk sex in significantly larger numbers than their elders. Studies suggest young gays are more likely to have had multiple partners and unprotected anal intercourse, the two leading risk factors for HIV infection in the past twelve months. In the San Francisco area, a Department of Health survey indicated that a second wave of HIV/AIDS infections is taking shape, with the highest incidence among gay men between seventeen and twenty-five years. According to the Centers for Disease Control and Prevention, diagnosed cases of AIDS among gay men from thirteen to twenty-nine crept upward last year, in defiance of the overall downward trend.

HIV/AIDS'S EFFECT ON THE COMMUNITIES LEAST ABLE TO DEAL WITH IT

According to a recent report by the National Research Council, the AIDS epidemic is "settling into spatially and socially isolated groups and possibly becoming endemic in them." To find those at risk for HIV/AIDS, the report went on, one need only look at where bacterial and sexually transmitted diseases (STDs) are epidemic—"zones of urban poverty, poor health, drug addiction and social disintegration."

Sexually transmitted diseases are again becoming epidemic. The number of reported cases of chancroid, once almost unknown in the United States, has increased sevenfold over the past decade. An estimated four million Americans suffer from chlamydia, and each year there are between 200,000 and 500,000 new cases of genital herpes. Between 1984 and 1990, the time HIV began to spread significantly from white gay communities into communities of color, the number of cases of syphilis for African-American males almost tripled. The number of new cases among African-American women in that same period almost quadrupled. These statistics chart the future course of HIV. And if we are to intervene effectively in this trend as health educators, we must not make the same mistakes that were made with regard to public education around the spread of STDs in the African-American community. We must not fall prey to "blaming the victim," in this case African-American women, for not embracing a message of self-protection when the problem was likely in how the message was imparted and in the mistaken assumption that everyone has the same resources available to support healthy practices.

While every one of the sexually transmitted diseases that has been mentioned is treatable and in most cases curable, this country's poorest neighborhoods, where these diseases are concentrated, are faced with a decaying public-health infrastructure that once existed to detect and treat STDs. The government today spends 23 percent less (in constant dollars) on controlling STDs than it did in 1950.

Reversing this slide has to be a priority of any revitalized HIV/ AIDS prevention strategy. According to the Coalition on STDs, a group of public-health organizations, this would probably require adding about $110 million to the Centers for Disease Control's current STD budget of $90 million. Considering that the direct and indirect costs of HIV and AIDS in the United States in 1992 amounted to $64 billion, that seems like a small price to pay.

We must stress that it is specific behaviors that put people, or some groups, at risk. Groups, particularly ethnic groups, should not be viewed as risk categories in and of themselves. Communities of color are diverse and heterogeneous. Yet the culture and social context of those at risk must be examined and messages designed in a cultural language to assist the processing of information received.

Culture comprises complex sets of behaviors and social norms. Who we are is often what we do. Therefore, asking people to change what they do can often imply far more that simply changing a behavior; it can be interpreted as asking people to change who they are.

Although it is specific behaviors that put people at risk, there is a case to be made for providing extra funding to target racial and ethnic groups. The recent report by the National Commission on AIDS states that African-Americans and Latinos make up 46 percent of all the AIDS cases in the United States, which is disproportionate to their representation in the general population. The report then argues that the disease should be treated as a racial issue. "Racial inequality in the U.S.," the report reads, "is pre-eminent among festering social problems . . . upon which the epidemic feeds."

Poverty, homelessness, unemployment, lack of access to medical care—all of the social ills of our times—contribute to the likelihood that HIV, like a host of other social problems, will settle in those communities with the fewest defenses. Communities without the infrastructure to provide even the most basic protection to their members need special attention.

TARGETING AIDS EDUCATION

These are the days of tight budgets—at the federal, state, and local levels. There simply is not enough money to provide unlimited HIV/AIDS education equally to all segments of the population. In California, for example, state funds for AIDS prevention and education declined between 1989 and 1993, while the number of AIDS cases and risk groups have grown.

Realistically, shrinking dollars means education and prevention efforts must be targeted to those people most at risk. The interventions must also be culturally appropriate and as effective as possible. HIV/AIDS education and prevention programs must be cost effective. A 1993 University of California at San Francisco report stated that for each new infection averted, the state would save approximately $100,000 in lifetime AIDS treatment costs and $10,000 annually in HIV treatment costs.

AIDS education should be focused, and any focused attack on the spread of HIV should involve behavioral modification. Think, for example, what could be done with New York City's injection drug users, 50 percent of whom are now infected. Because of that extraordinarily high rate of infection, this group is a principal point of entry of HIV into the younger heterosexual population. Intravenous heroin users, however, are an easily identifiable group. A relatively small proportion are younger than thirty. One AIDS prevention strategy, according to Des Jarlais, may consist of no more than this: telling teenagers and young adults in Harlem, Washington Heights, and the Bronx not to have sex with people more than a few years older than themselves, thereby cutting the connection between heroin users and the younger generation. This may not seem as effective as telling young people to wear a condom, but then again, it is advice that may be followed.

Sometimes the risk behaviors or risk routes are somewhat circuitous, and need to be taken into account when targeting education and prevention efforts. For instance, researchers have recently identified alcohol as one potential cause of sexual risk taking. The link between alcohol and sexual behavior appears to be a matter of consensus. A small but growing body of literature provides support for an association between drinking and risky sex, although whether there is a causal link between the two remains unclear. Nevertheless, it may be important to take alcohol into account in some AIDS education and prevention programs. As Lynn Cooper points out, "By identifying individual, sociocultural, and situational variables that moderate the impact of alcohol on sexual risk behaviors, we may more effectively target high-risk groups and high-risk situations."

It is thus essential to conduct AIDS education and prevention by targeting those people most at risk. This perspective is reinforced by a 1993 report on the California State Office of AIDS, written by researchers from the Institute of Health Policy Studies at the University of California at San Francisco. One of the key findings was that too much of the state's money is being spent to educate the general public and too little is spent on those populations most heavily impacted by HIV. Funding decisions have become political footballs, and often politics rather than sound health policy determines where the money goes.

There have been some small strides in this area. During the early years of the U.S. Conference of Mayors' CDC grants, projects were funded to educate the general population and men who have sex with other men. During the last few years, however, funding priorities have refocused on organizations treating minority populations, with efforts such as teen theater for Hispanic youths in East Los Angeles and peer-group education for African-American gays in Detroit. Seed funding provided by the grants program for CBOs has supported the development of creative, often novel approaches to reaching target populations. Further funding is needed to reach other underserved groups, from the mentally ill to migrant farm workers to homeless persons to street youths to incarcerated populations, to name but a few.

There are also groups that may not necessarily be at high risk but are difficult to reach through traditional health education channels, and less is known about their HIV/AIDS knowledge and behaviors. Recent immigrants, nonliterate individuals, and non–English speakers are only a few examples of such groups.

Finally, we must begin to realize that prevention education does not take place within a vacuum; that there are social, political, and cultural barriers that also impact health educators' abilities to function effectively, many of which are beyond the control of health educators but continue to inhibit the efficacy of prevention education in the United States. Among these are the following:

Insufficient Emphasis on Risk Assessments It is of great concern that, at this stage in the epidemic, there is insufficient targeting of those individuals at highest risk of HIV. It is time to acknowledge that those at highest risk of infection need more than "one-shot" interventions; that long-term prevention education with repeated interventions may be necessary to help these individuals change their high risk behaviors. Conversely, there is limited utility in focusing limited resources on providing basic HIV/AIDS information to those at minimal risk of infection (many of whom are already aware of the information), or to continue merely passing out bleach and condoms to individuals without the skills to implement the requisite behavior change. This is not to imply that we should allocate resources only to easily identified or affected communities—epidemiological data should be made available and used not only to look at where the epidemic has been, but also where it is going.

Insufficient Emphasis on Skills Development with Those at Highest Risk While the actions needed to prevent HIV infection are relatively simple, many individuals lack the skills needed to effectively implement the necessary sexual or needle-using practices or to overcome cultural or gender bias. Women continue to be victims of economic, social, and political bias, including the arena of sexual politics for women. For example, despite the supposed "liberation" of women, women continue to face substantive cultural taboos against their active participation in sexual negotiations; they are often viewed as "overly aggressive," "unfeminine," and so forth when they try to assert themselves in or control sexual negotiations. Many women, fearing sexual rejection, are unable to take control of their sexual lives. Too often excluded from the decision of *when* to have sex, they are often also excluded from decisions about *how* to have sex (e.g., whether to use a condom); and are forced into sexual relationships that reenact cultural norms rather than directly confronting those norms, acting in their own self-interest, and perhaps saving their lives.

Lack of Understanding of Cultural Determinants Affecting HIV Prevention and Care While there are numerous references in the health-education literature describing the need to provide AIDS education within a cultural context, all too often health educators overlook the cultural determinants of the populations they are trying to reach. They do not engage in the necessary study of a given culture or are unwilling or unable to hire staff from the impacted communities, and are therefore unaware of the appropriate "message," the "messenger," and the population's experience of the dominant culture. Meaning is culturally derived, and we cannot develop culturally appropriate health-education messages without understanding those cultures we are trying to impact.

Categorical Funding Streams Health educators increasingly agree there is a need to approach HIV prevention education within the larger context of health promotion and wellness in order to more accurately reflect the way people live their lives. Prevention education should be more encompassing and comprehensive, dealing with a number of topics related to good health. Even federal funding initiatives require grant applicants to engage in cross-agency collaborations; however, in truth, there is little collaboration at the federal level. Categorical funding streams reflect continued competition among federal agencies and create substantive barriers to the actual delivery of holistic health promotion.

Competition for Funding In far too many instances, the gay community has been pitted against communities of color and forced to compete for limited prevention funding. Ironically, rather than celebrating gains in the slowing of infections rates, these communities are forced to flaunt or even inflate their HIV infection rates in hopes of acquiring needed funding. We need to stop viewing AIDS funding as a zero-sum game, with winners and losers. Instead, we need to adopt a strategy of interdependence—believing that how we deal with one another will ultimately reflect on our success at stopping the spread of HIV in all communities.

Lack of Communication and Collaboration between Academic Researchers and Prevention Educators While both university researchers and prevention educators are working diligently to stop the spread of HIV, all too often they work in parallel (and never intersecting) tracks. Prevention educators often identify with the communities in which they work and tend to distrust academic researchers. They often see researchers as "opportunists" who "suck data out of their communities" but rarely share their findings with the impacted community—that their expertise is not valued by the academic research community. Conversely, researchers often complain about educators' tendencies to inappropriately project anecdotal data findings across populations. It is clear that both sides have legitimate concerns about the other, but, at this point in time, we cannot afford to point fingers; rather we need to begin to develop a dialogue, communicate effectively with one another, and enter into respectful collaborations designed to slow the spread of HIV.

AN OVERVIEW OF THIS BOOK

This book is designed to get the attention of health educators, researchers, and policymakers—to challenge the current "state of the art" with regard to HIV prevention education and to highlight the work of just a few of the many dedicated, pioneering health educators working to stop the spread of HIV.

For many individuals who have been identified as difficult to reach or at increased risk of HIV infection, special approaches are needed to intervene successfully in the spread of HIV/AIDS. The chapters in this book describe these approaches, based on the authors' work in a variety of communities and with different high-risk target populations.

This book is about what works now. The book describes how to tailor HIV education and prevention efforts to specific communities, including how to identify those most at risk, what types of interventions are most appropriate to those communities, how to "engage" those most at risk, and the role of participatory evaluation in determining the effectiveness of community education efforts.

For at least the next several years, the most effective strategies for stemming the spread of HIV infection are education of the public and voluntary changes in behavior. There are many social ills for which public education is prescribed as a cure, especially where there are few specific responses available. Education can sometimes be a soft substitute for hard action. Yet public education about HIV infection will continue to be a critical public-health measure, even if a vaccine or drug becomes available. Education in this instance is not only the transfer of knowledge, but has the added dimension of inducing, persuading, and otherwise motivating people to avoid the transmission of HIV.

If behavior modification is the goal of education about HIV/AIDS, the content of the material presented must address the behavior in question as directly as possible. Educators must be prepared to speak plainly about the sexual practices that put people at risk of infection. Furthermore, they must understand that behavior change must be addressed within a cultural context if real, long-term changes in behavior are to occur. Moreover, health educators must not adopt the same reductionist line when thinking about culture as that used when thinking about the behaviors they so enthusiastically encourage. Culture and subculture are multifaceted and complex arenas, and effective approaches to prevention education must grapple with this complexity. For example, in dealing with injection drug users, the obstacles to educational success include both the attitudes of users and the laws that affect their conduct (both of which are culturally based). And while research demonstrates that many injection drug users have changed their needle-using behaviors, far fewer have adopted safe sex practices.

The most obvious targets for education are presently identified high-risk groups: gay men, IDUs, prostitutes, people who have multiple sexual partners, and sexual partners of those in high-risk groups. Although gays, especially in urban areas, are frequently portrayed as highly organized and easily reached, it would be a mistake to assume that all men who have sex with other men perceive themselves as belonging to the gay community, read the gay press, or listen to gay leaders. Many rural gays or gay ethnic minorities are not identified with the urban white gay culture.

While the HIV epidemic affects all segments of society, it is important to recognize that each distinct segment has its own unique educational needs. The National AIDS Commission recognizes that it is behavior, not membership in a particular group, that places a person at risk of HIV infection. However, the educational response to the epidemic needs to acknowledge the eclectic nature of our society and effectively match the educational approach with a receptive target population. It is time to realize that, although the content of the message may be the same, a variety of voices are needed to communicate that message.

2

Successes and Failures in the Gay Community: HIV Prevention Workshops at Gay Men's Health Crisis

James M. Holmes and
Steven Humes

HIV prevention efforts among gay men are at a critical juncture. While annual seroconversions among urban gay men declined significantly in the mid-1980s, recent reports of a "second wave" of HIV infection have raised serious questions about the efficacy of existing prevention programs (Gross, 1993). Studies conducted in urban areas also suggest that gay men are experiencing acute emotional distress that affects their ability to practice risk reduction consistently. Psychological symptoms such as social isolation, depression, anxiety disorders, adjustment disorders, post-traumatic stress syndrome, hypochondriasis, and sexual dysfunction have been noted (Odets, 1990); studies in New York point to similar problems in their samples of gay men (Martin, 1988; Tross, 1986). A 1993 San Francisco survey found a number of factors that tended to presage incidents of unsafe behavior, including feelings of grief and loss, low self-esteem, societal homophobia, hopelessness about the future, survivor guilt, a tenuous connection to the gay community, and feelings of inevitability about contracting HIV (Communication Technologies, 1993).

AIDS educators contend with growing feelings of inadequacy as they face an epidemic that defies efforts at control, while the precipitating social and psychological factors seem to grow more complex with time. In this chapter, we will examine some of the assumptions, both explicit and implicit, underlying prevention efforts with gay men to date. As an example, a review of some of the AIDS prevention workshops of Gay Men's Health Crisis, one large urban community-based organization, will be undertaken to illuminate some of the strengths and shortcomings of this approach.

Gay Men's Health Crisis (GMHC), the first organization to acknowledge and address AIDS, has provided prevention services to gay men in New York City since the beginning of the epidemic. These services, which vary in content and structure, have been largely intended to influence gay men to adopt and maintain safer sexual practices which will, in turn, reduce their risk for HIV infection. While a range of educational techniques have been employed toward this end, this chapter will highlight the experiential workshops developed by GMHC since 1985. They have been the centerpiece of GMHC's AIDS prevention model, and while they have been adapted and embellished, the model remains one standard for AIDS prevention work among gay men, as well as among other populations. It is our belief that, while GMHC has been largely successful in its prevention efforts, these workshops have sometimes overlooked or misjudged the social and psychological realities of gay men, and consequently have compounded the difficulties that may be primary precipitators of unsafe sex among them.

In April 1985, GMHC undertook the "800 Men Study" to compare three models of AIDS prevention for gay men. One model used relatively traditional didactic techniques with the primary function of giving information, including medical and scientific information, and little effort was made to reduce anxiety through avoiding negative or fear-inducing messages. A second model used more experiential techniques, including workshops, and emphasized explicit, erotic, or sex-affirming language and visual materials. A third model paralleled the second, but included only erotic language and no visual material. The study itself was fraught with methodological difficulties, but the research team concluded that a combination of didactic content, experiential learning, and verbal and visual erotic material seemed to enhance individuals' ability to practice safer sex. The conceptual framework for these conclusions revolved around two hypotheses. One involved the method of education, contending that experiential learning would be more effective in AIDS prevention than didactic learning. The other involved the content of that education, asserting that explicit visual and verbal erotic material would facilitate more effective change among gay men. Although the research methods have been questioned and the conclusions, therefore, challenged, these two assumptions implicit in the 800 Men Study have guided prevention efforts at GMHC and elsewhere.

In development at the same time, and used as one of the experiential portions of the 800 Men Study, was what has become known as "Eroticizing Safer Sex" (ESS). In a retrospective article (Shernoff and Bloom, 1991), the surviving author of this workshop postulated that difficulties in modifying sexual behaviors arose from a variety of issues, including (1) confusion about what behaviors were indeed risky, (2) anger at having to change long-established behaviors, (3) internalized homophobia or erotophobia, (4) denial of risk, and (5) a sense that HIV could not be avoided. ESS sought to provide a forum where gay men could receive information about safer-sex behaviors and gain practice in negotiating them, yet also have an opportunity to discuss their emotional responses to the epidemic in a structured, sex-positive environment. In conceptualizing their workshop in this fashion, the authors acknowledged an important additional component of successful behavior change—group interaction. By creating a space for participants to explore their feelings and values in relation to others, they set up an environment in which group norms could begin to be modified and mutual support for behavior change could develop.

Shernoff and Bloom, while facilitating Eroticizing Safer Sex workshops from 1985 to 1987, heard participants frequently say that while they understood how to make safer sex more erotic, they needed help in learning how to meet men in nonsexual ways and court them. Whereas sexual encounters prior to the advent of AIDS had often been anonymous, the threat of HIV transmission made it more important to discuss the way men related to one another both sexually and nonsexually. This socialization deficit led to the creation in 1988 of a second workshop, "Men Meeting Men" (MMM), wherein the socialization context and skills of the participants were the focus. The authors labeled this a "second-generation intervention." The first-generation interventions, in a sense, inform participants of the facts of safer sex and help them to make certain changes in their attitudes about sex. The second-generation interventions help participants explore what it means to put these new behaviors into practice.

As this new workshop was increasingly offered, the authors noted a particular problem in the structure of ESS and MMM. Dividing sexual and relationship issues through separate workshops reinforced a split between sexuality and intimacy that had historically been a therapeutic issue for the men whom the authors had seen in their private practices. A third workshop, "Sex, Dating and Intimacy" (SDI), was thus designed as a day-long amalgamation of the prior two interventions.

Finally, in 1992, after a barrage of reports about what has commonly been called "relapse," a day-long workshop called "Keep It Up" was developed. This workshop helped men look at how they assess risk; examined the role of peer norms and stress in safer-sex practices; helped men analyze barriers to safer sex and triggers for unsafe sex, and explored ways of coping with those triggers; and attempted to build the confidence and commitments to safer sex of participants (Miller et al., 1993).

The surviving author of ESS, MMM, and SDI has described the assumptions and values that underlayed their thinking. Some of these assumptions are the following:

1. The workshops are designed to help people recognize and tolerate the feelings, sometimes intense, which arise when involved in negotiations surrounding sexual decisions and activities. Being able to act on sexual feelings is one indication of a healthy, well integrated individual.

2. The workshops are intended to be sex-positive. That is, they recognize the negative effects of "abstinence only" and other messages with heavy moral tones, and emphasize that sexual expression is a normal part of a healthy life.

3. Since alcohol and drugs are strong behavior disinhibitors, effective ways of dealing with the anxiety that often arises from social encounters without resorting to substance use is an important workshop component.

4. Positive self-esteem is a prerequisite for the adoption of risk-reduction behaviors. Only by valuing oneself can one be concerned about one's own safety or the safety of one's partner; therefore, esteem-enhancing interventions must be part of the workshops. This includes, especially, a positive value placed on homosexuality.

5. The diversity of sexual behavior, from one-night stands to committed relationships, must be accepted in the workshops. The right of the individual to express his sexual needs in his own way, the authors maintain, has been at the heart of the gay liberation struggle and is the basis for "self-respect and pride."

6. Safer-sex interventions are a form of community organizing in that they strengthen bonds between affiliated members and promote community responsibility and pride. Joseph et al. (1987) and Prieur (1990) found that gay men who lacked a social network and supporting environment were more likely to engage in unprotected sex.

7. The workshops not only help participants adopt safer-sex behaviors, they aim to help people consistently maintain them.

Owing to inadequate or nonexistent evaluation of these workshops, any discussion of their success is largely conjecture. Save for Keep It Up, which has been systematically evaluated, impact objectives for the other workshops have not been adequately formulated in order for measurement to occur, and systematic evaluations have not yet been attempted. Although the workshops still draw large numbers of people, it is still mostly unknown why they come and how they have been changed, if at all, as a result of the workshop experience. It is expected that some people may attend workshops because they afford opportunities to meet other men, others because they want to build skills around safer-sex practices (Humes and Waters, 1992). Although both may be important factors in attracting men to the workshops and facilitating their adoption of safer behaviors, little is understood still about the exact relationship between motivation to attend safe-sex workshops and successful behavior change, so that adequate measurement of workshop effectiveness remains to be done. However, even within this framework, it is possible to make some observations about factors that should be considered when further refining AIDS prevention workshops for gay men.

As our understanding has evolved, successive workshops have increasingly acknowledged a more complex social and psychological context that must be addressed if effective behavior change is to take place. To meet this emerging awareness, a number of changes in the workshops have been made. The workshops have grown longer to allow for more in-depth exploration of complex issues. They attempt to integrate the issues into a greater whole, as, for instance, in SDI, which connects the need for negotiation skills with the need to meet and socialize with other men, or Keep It Up, which connects personal risk assessment with stress and lack of confidence to practice safer sex. At the same time, there has been a recently growing awareness of the precursors to unsafe sex, but workshops still have not fully capitalized on this greater understanding. For although there is a better understanding of the motivators for risky behaviors, and a consequent ability to manipulate these motivators to allow for less risky options, several primary issues have still not been dealt with adequately by AIDS educators who operate the AIDS prevention programs targeting gay men.

We have divided our discussion of these issues into two categories: (1) how gay male sexuality and its context has been conceptualized and guides GMHC's (and, needless to say, other organizations') AIDS prevention efforts, and (2) the methods employed to achieve particular behavioral or attitudinal ends.

In examining the construction of homosexual sexuality, it is useful to consider the assumptions about the population for whom the programs have been designed and whom they are trying to reach. The stated target audience for all of the GMHC workshops has been self-identified gay or bisexual men, with the exception of Keep It Up, which targets only gay men. Without questioning too deeply what "gay" and "bisexual" may have meant to the participants, the workshops forged ahead in the early 1980s, unaware of the deep consequences of the assumptions the workshop designers had made. As Kayal (1993) notes, the 800 Men Project "supposed a universal type of gay sexuality, disregarding an individual's social class, education, religious beliefs, and ethnic background." For early AIDS prevention efforts for gay men, sex was considered unidimensionally, that is, as a singular phenomenon which occurred in a context that mirrored that of the predominantly white, middle-class, educated gay men who designed the interventions. The urban gay "clone," as described by Levine (1979), in reality reflects only a narrow slice of the continuum of gay male experience. By positing such a cookie-cutter notion of gay male sexuality, the AIDS prevention workshops deny the diversity of male sexual experience. As prevention efforts began to diversify, that context began to be challenged and, gradually, grew more complex. Yet the conceptualization of sex has remained unidimensional. And the prevention efforts to date have been largely advertised for "gay and bisexual men," whether the potential consumer perceives himself as labeled in that manner or labeled at all according to a sexual orientation or identity.

Alfred Kinsey's groundbreaking studies of homosexuality in the 1940s described sexual "preference" on a seven-point continuum, from "no overt" to "exclusively" homosexual experience; reporting on actual history of sexual practice, as opposed to fantasy or dream life (Masters and Johnson, 1979). A more recent study has reported that 20 percent of American males have homosexual impulses, even though many do not act on these impulses (Sirica, 1994). AIDS prevention educators, likewise, must explore their understanding of homosexuality and apply that greater understanding to the practice of AIDS prevention for their target audience. In fact, the construct "sexual preference" can be conceptualized as a matrix of interrelated dimensions, each impacting upon the other to describe the meanings of sexual life and experience to the individual. Primary dimensions are orientation, identity, and behavior. All of these, it seems, have great importance for not only the contact and recruitment of consumers for prevention efforts, but how the consumers accept and integrate the prevention work done with and for them. Health education theorists state that successful behavior-change programs consider the context and meaning of behaviors for the individual and plan programs to address those behaviors within their appropriate context.

The first dimension is sexual orientation, that which determines attraction to the same or opposite gender. Regardless of the various debates concerning the etiology of homosexual orientation, most theorists posit a range of orientation potential among humans, leaving to further study the arguments about how fixed or fluid that orientation may be for any individual at any point in time or throughout the lifespan. For those who have or expect that they might have an orientation that deviates from the so-called societal norm of heterosexuality, regardless of where they fall on the behavior spectrum, they may not identify with the labels "gay" or "bisexual" or "men who have sex with men," which are commonly applied to them and which may exclude them from the very prevention efforts supposedly targeted specifically to them. At the same time, their fantasy life will most likely contain thoughts of how they would be perceived by others if others were to know about their deviation. This couples orientation directly with identity.

Sexual identity has both public and private facets. The private includes personal thoughts, dreams, and fantasies and is the seat of great fear and expectation for many gay men. Having neither general societal acceptance nor adequate positive role models often leaves them unwilling or unable to acknowledge their desire to engage in behaviors that might put them at risk for HIV. For some, the fear is so powerful it is immobilizing, causing a self-imposed prohibition of all sexual activity on the one hand, or a denial of the activity that does occur, on the other.

The public facet includes the willingness or ability to allow others to know about the private identity. For many men, to "come out" has become a rite of passage into a happier, albeit controversial, position about public acknowledgment of private beliefs and behaviors. Many more, those to whom the labels "gay" or "bisexual" may not appeal, must deal with their fears, which include the risk of uncomfortable public identity.

Ultimately, it is sexual behaviors that put one at risk for HIV infection. Early on in AIDS prevention it became accepted practice, in order to soften the stigma associated with AIDS, that educators would address risk in terms of behaviors, instead of group identifications. While this has been an important tool for circumventing attempts by some to avoid awareness of their risk, it has largely made invisible the dimensions of orientation and identity that bear such great personal meaning to individuals. It is our contention that men (or women and children, for that matter) who are at risk do not conceptualize their risk in terms of "behaviors," but rather in terms of more personal meanings the individual attributes, either consciously or unconsciously, to these behaviors. Behaviors-only conceptualizations deny the relational aspects of human sexual interaction. Public health is interested in the behaviors; the individual is interested in the meanings of those behaviors and the impact of potential disruption of patterns of established behavior.

Appropriate attention to the relation aspects of sexual interaction must include discussion of the purpose of the behaviors under discussion. In an atmosphere of erotophobia and homophobia, it is easy to pass moral judgments about behaviors that may lead to negative consequences. These attacks come not only from outside the community. As Kayal (1993) states,

Sex for its own sake cannot be the basis for either AIDS prevention, group solidarity, or politicization. When mutuality, concern, and compassion are missing from human relationships, the fabric and basis of community are damaged, the politicization process is undermined, and social or institutional change retarded. From the perspective of community, what really matters is the quality of gay relations, not the quantity. Basically, choosing multiple and anonymous sex partners is a function of self-image and reflects powerlessness and fatalism.

While building esteem is an important function of AIDS prevention, harsh criticisms of sexual practices, however unpopular these practices may be among the larger society, serve only to undermine the self-image and power of gay men. Kayal takes a position not uncommon, even within the gay community, which neglects to acknowledge the varied purposes of sexual activity among people and situations. The confusion of sexual activity within relationships denies that they are two distinct and independently functioning things. The same individual may have relationships of consequence with or without sexual contact. During the same period but under different circumstances the same person may engage in sexual activity that expressly avoids significant or emotional involvement. The two situations may coexist independently or coincidentally

(McWhirter and Mattison, 1984). To address AIDS prevention efforts to only one or the other is to deny reality and to do an incomplete job. To use AIDS prevention messages to moralize about sexual practices is phobic and damaging to the effort. Shernoff and Bloom's (1991) acknowledgment of the variability of sexual behavior takes this into account, but still may not provide adequate support for sorting out the confusions the individual feels as he experiences the social messages he receives, as well as grapples with his own understanding of the meanings he attributes to the various behaviors and contexts for those behaviors as he experiences them.

Beyond the misunderstanding of sexual preference, there has been an incomplete conceptualization of the precursors to unsafe sex; tending to view the problem in the "here and now" and failing to note some of the developmental antecedents that impact upon gay men.

There are a number of developmental issues particular to gay men. Chief among them is coming out. Of the various models developed to explain this process, most propose a division between private and public aspects of coming out (McWhirter and Mattison, 1984). The private aspect has to do with the individual's awareness of his orientation and his developing comfort with and conscious acknowledgment to himself of that orientation. The public aspect deals with awareness, comfort, and conscious acokwledgment, but among people associated with the individual; first close friends and family members, then expanding to larger circles of association. Because of the discrepant and sometimes conflicting agendas at various stages of life and between the private and public aspects of coming out, gay men often learn to survive by tolerating a great deal of discomfort regarding very personal thoughts, feelings, and behaviors. Or they learn to deny these thoughts, feelings, and behaviors altogether. This learned ability to separate whole parts of one's life from other parts can lead to confusion about how to behave in different circumstances and, therefore, may leave men highly vulnerable to risk, yet unaware of that risk. Inability to feel comfortable, either publicly or privately, with one's homosexual orientation can force one, in essence, to "live a lie" which, in turn, can be detrimental to prevention efforts. Prevention models that do not take this into account miss an important opportunity.

Tied to this are various additional discrepancies that distance gay men from other people, causing possible relationship difficulties, or from themselves, nurturing denial. The "heterosexual assumption" imposed upon most gay men, the fact that they are raised by parents who are different from them in critical ways, and the fact that their environments give them few positive models to emulate all present developmental burdens that need to be addressed before prevention efforts can be effective. All of the above contribute, as well, to a possible delayed adolescence in which sexual experimentation, dating behavior, and exploration of relationships may be postponed far later than that of heterosexual people, leaving the gay person ready to begin these activities in a discordant position. Societal expectations of performance for a person in his twenties or thirties are far different from those of a teenager, even if the older person is first facing typically teenage issues.

Finally, of great importance to gay men in the 1990s is the effect of the AIDS epidemic itself on development and passage through the lifespan. The assumptions made about gay men in the early 1980s, however inappropriate then, are clearly less accurate today. AIDS has substantially changed the gay community. It is the norm for many in this community to experience shortened life-expectancy for themselves or for those around them. Grief, loss, blaming, societal homophobia—as well as a stronger community connection for some—all serve to separate gay men's lives from the larger society even more strikingly today than at the beginning of the epidemic. HIV infection itself, as a demographic characteristic, splits the gay community in two. All these factors have critical importance to current AIDS prevention efforts. The lives of gay men have clearly taken on new meaning since the advent of AIDS.

How this relates to the workshop methods in use for prevention is interesting. The GMHC workshops have always relied on cognitive–behavioral models. Whereas they have employed the latest of techniques, these techniques may not be the most effective choices to address complex material. Some of the broad goals which Shernoff and Bloom have articulated cannot be supported in workshops of relatively brief duration and which exclusively employ structured experiential exercises. Structured learning assumes that information brought to conscious awareness will, with the building or strengthening of specific skills, precipitate a desired attitudinal or behavioral outcome. Whereas exercises may be useful in helping participants understand and integrate information about or awareness of their own situations, many of the complex developmental concerns listed will only be resolved by a repeated "working through" process. An event which takes into account the less conscious aspects of motivation may be more appropriate. Working through such issues also requires more time than the typical workshop allows.

Associated with this is the assumption that "triggers" for unsafe sex, such as being drunk or high, being overwhelmed by the attractiveness of one's partner or the heat of the moment, and so forth, can be overcome by cognition and skills building. While they may be superficially the same from one individual to another, they remain only triggers, and the true motivators for the unsafe behaviors are more likely a multiplicity of less conscious impulses that emanate from experiences unique to each individual. We have found that skills-building exercises alone may be ineffective in resolving developmental conflicts of long standing. Also, as has been suggested, sexual behavior is so intimately tied to one's conceptions of orientation and identity that building self-efficacy around handling triggers to unsafe sex may be only a small part of the overall task.

It is now arguable whether ESS, MMM, and SDI can accomplish all of the authors' goals, even as they were originally conceptualized, using only a cognitive–behavioral model. For example, while it is true that self-esteem is associated with the ability to practice safer sex, it is unlikely that a workshop can do more than begin to help participants clarify their self-esteem issues. Certainly, coming together as a group has its positive effects: Hearing similar stories, participating in common activities, and experiencing others' achievements all contribute to a stronger sense of self and a stronger community. However, self-esteem is variable and multidetermined. Group pride can support positive self-esteem; it cannot replace individual lack of self-worth, a product of years of social conditioning. The value of a self-esteem exercise seems more symbolic than real unless it occurs in the context of a longer discussion or format that addresses developmental issues.

Likewise, the workshop approach to sustained change is faulty. The curricula tend to see behavior change as an either/or proposition, and not something with which one must grapple on a day-to-day-basis. Since there appears to be no acceptable rate of HIV seroconversion in the gay community, it has led to the message that no lapse from stringent safer-sex guidelines is to be tolerated. There is no room for error; only stark success or utter failure. Implicit is the message that gay men who are unable to practice safer sex consistently are morally and psychologically defective. Odets (1994) has suggested that by declaring one should use a condom each and every time one has sex, unprotected sex is stigmatized, thus making it more difficult to acknowledge and to alter. Although the workshops currently give individuals the opportunity to mourn lost behaviors, they are not yet a safe forum for someone to admit practicing unsafe behaviors for whatever reason.

A "harm reduction" model, on the other hand, assumes that participants may lapse into old behaviors and, if so, will need assistance in resetting goals and re-establishing their new behaviors.

Interventions employing such models typically require sustained contact with the target audience in order to increase the likelihood of their success. For example, a recently implemented GMHC program entitled "Steps toward Change" places HIV positive men who are having difficulty changing destructive alcohol or drug use behaviors into a small group for a ten-week period and works with them to establish reasonable goals for change. This realistic approach was lacking in the earlier GMHC workshops in relation to both substance use *and* sexual behavior.

Finally, while it is true that safer-sex workshops serve a community organizing function by strengthening bonds between affiliated members and promoting community responsibility and pride, it is undoubtedly the case that men who attend the workshops already possess some sense of affiliation with the gay community and must already be invested in behavior change (Prochaska et al., 1992), or they would not be there. Those most "at risk"—the unaffiliated or disinterested—must be the target of a more complex effort at community mobilization than has heretofore occurred, in order to bring them to the point of considering changing their behavior.

Given our critique of the early GMHC workshops, it is important to keep in mind that these early efforts were pioneering at their time. For, as is well known, seroconversions among gay men dropped dramatically in the mid-1980s. This may seem surprising, except that, after all, those who did the earliest work were members of the population most at risk. (Many have since succumbed to AIDS themselves.) Therefore, there was little need to analyze the meanings of the behaviors that put them at risk. They, as their own target population, knew inherently who and what they were dealing with. This is what makes AIDS such a unique phenomenon in the history of public health: The population initially most severely affected defined itself by the very factors that placed its members most at risk. In the post-Stonewall 1970s, the newly liberated gay community prided itself on an identity that was based in its sexual expression, and when AIDS arrived on the scene it was only a short step to educate those who considered themselves a part of this community to the necessity for adjustments in behaviors that, after all, were publicly discussed and displayed as a part of a cultural identity. This made possible the sweeping behavior changes that have been classed as among the most dramatic in public-health history.

These dramatic changes, however, lulled AIDS educators and program planners into the belief that their work had been easy and was largely over, without the understanding that those community members with whom they had been seemingly successful were the highly motivated minority and that the majority of gay men had not been "reached" or that the task of changing their behaviors was far from complete. In order to effectively plan such a program, a concerted diagnosis of the social, behavioral, and environmental factors that influence the behavior would first be necessary (Green and Kreuter, 1991). In the early 1980s, AIDS was not considered a long-range health issue; the crisis was immediate and overwhelming. The activists who did the first AIDS prevention work were not trained in health education and there seemed little time to analyze all of the social and psychological factors that contributed to the situation that needed to be addressed.

Consequently, early AIDS prevention programs, including those at Gay Men's Health Crisis and elsewhere, did not take sufficiently into account the complexities of identity and culture for their population. Over time, the programs grew less successful as they exhaused the most motivated segments of their populations—those most similar to the intitial educators—and tried to address those men who comprised the majority of those needing behavior-change interventions. Sadly, with such seeming initial success, energies and resources for AIDS prevention soon shifted away from gay men to other groups considered "harder to reach." Interestingly, it has been largely accepted that the models developed for gay men would not be adequate for these other populations, and models have been and are being developed which do take into consideration the complex contextual millieu of those populations in order to assure the greatest success. Now targeting audiences that are harder to reach, AIDS prevention workshops for other than the gay men who did the initial AIDS prevention work are being designed to accommodate the subtleties in their identities and contexts. In fact, the term "hard-to-reach" may be nothing more than a euphemism for the toil it takes the educator to assess and understand a community before designing an intervention. An adequate assessment of the initial gay men who were recipients of AIDS prevention workshops was never done. It was almost serendipitous that the programs worked at all—but highly lucky that they worked as well as they did.

REFERENCES

Communication Technologies. (1993). *A Call of a New Generation of AIDS Prevention for Gay and Bisexual Men in San Francisco.* San Francisco: Communication Technologies.

Green, L., and M. Kreuter. (1991). *Health Promotion Planing: An Educational and Environmental Approach.* Mountain View, Calif.: Mayfield.

Gross, J. (1993). "Second Wave of AIDS Feared by Officials in San Francisco." *The New York Times,* 11 December, pp. 1, 8.

Humes, S., and M. Waters. (1992). A Process Evaluation of "Eroticizing Safer Sex." Unpublished.

Joseph, J., S. Montgomery, J. Kirscht, R. Kessler, D. Ostrow, D. Emmons, and J. Phair. (1987). Perceived Risk of AIDS: Assessing the Behavioral and Psychosocial Consequences in a Cohort of Gay Men. *Journal of Applied Social Psychology* 17(3): 231–250.

Kayal, P. (1993). "The Sociological Imagination in AIDS Prevention Education among Gay Men." *The Socal and Behavioral Aspects of AIDS. Advances in Medical Sociology* 3: 201–221.

Levine, M. (1979). *Gay Ghetto.* New York: Harper & Row.

Martin, J. (1988). Psychological Consequences of AIDS-Related Bereavement among Gay Men. *Journal of Consulting and Clinical Psychology* 56(6): 856–862.

Masters, W., and V. Johnson. (1979). *Homosexuality in Perspective.* New York: Bantam Books.

McWhirter, D., and A. Mattison. (1984). *The Male Couple: How Relationships Develop.* Englewood Cliffs, N.J.: Prentice-Hall.

Miller, R., K. Bratholt, R. Frederick, A. Grogan, B. Johnson, J. Kosciw, D. McDonagh, M. Manalansan, and A. Motta Moraes. (1993). *An Evaluation of the "Keep It Up!" Workshop and Support Groups: Final Report.* New York: Gay Men's Health Crisis.

Odets, W. (1990). The Homosexualization of AIDS. *FOCUS: A Guide to AIDS Research and Counseling* 5(11): 1–2.

Odets, W. (1994). AIDS Education and Harm Reduction for Gay Men: Psychological Approaches to the 21st Century. *AIDS and Public Policy Journal* 9(1): 1–20.

Prieur, A. (1990). Norwegian Gay Men: Reasons for Continued Practice of Unsafe Sex. *AIDS Education and Prevention: An Interdisciplinary Journal* 2(2): 109–115.

Prochaska, J., C. DiClemente, and J. Norcross. (1992). In Search of How People Change: Applications to Addictive Behaviors. *American Psychologist* 47(9): 1102–1113.

Shernoff, M., and D. J. Bloom. (1991). Designing Effective AIDS Prevention Workshops for Gay and Bisexual Men. *AIDS Education and Prevention* 3(1): 31–46.

Sirica, J. (1994). "Study: 20% of Adults have Gay Impulses." *New York Newsday,* 18 August.

Tross, S. (1986). Psychological Impact of AIDS Spectrum Disorders in New York City. Presentation at the American Psychological Association Annual Meeting, Washington, D.C.

3

Building a Proud Gay Identity: Adult Responsibility for Ending the Expanding HIV Epidemic among Gay Male Youth

Brian T. Byrnes

A PORTRAIT OF ADOLESCENT AIDS IN THE UNITED STATES

By the middle of 1995, almost 82,000 cases of AIDS had been diagnosed in people between the ages of twenty and twenty-nine. Since AIDS is a lagging indicator of HIV infections by ten years or more, most of these people were infected with HIV during adolescence.[1] Over half of these infections occurred during anal intercourse between two adolescent gay males. Of the approximately 2,000 AIDS cases diagnosed among adolescent males aged thirteen to nineteen, 37 percent were among adolescent males who have sex with other males (32%) or adolescent males who both have sex with other males and inject drugs (5%). Among black and Latino adult and adolescent males diagnosed with AIDS, 48 percent and 52 percent, respectively, were among men who had sex with men. Among white adult and adolescent males, the proportion of male-to-male AIDS cases is even higher, at 85 percent (CDC, 1995).

The picture of HIV infection is somewhat harder to paint, largely because of the lack of tracking of new infections among gay men. However, there are a few studies which give us a perspective on the magnitude of the emerging gay male AIDS epidemic. One in four new HIV infections occurs in people under the age of twenty-three (Rosenburg et al., 1994). One-quarter of all the young gay males seeking treatment at selected sexually transmitted disease clinics serving adolescents between 1988 and 1990 were infected with HIV. Among those clinics, there was a minimum rate of 4 percent and a maximum rate of 47 percent, which put the median rate at about 25 percent. That median is ten times that of the next highest risk group, young urban black males (Wendell et al., 1990). Among a group of 258 gay men between the ages of seventeen and twenty-five who were surveyed at gay night clubs in San Francisco, 12 percent tested HIV positive, with higher rates among those in the seventeen-to-nineteen and twenty-to-twenty-two-year-old age groups (14.3% and 14.0%, respectively). Among gay men of color, the rates were even higher (22.9% for African Americans and 14.3% for Latinos) (Lemp et al., 1994).

Unprotected anal intercourse with an infected partner accounts for the largest number of these new HIV infections, followed by sharing needles and "works" among injection drug–using gay youth. A survey of 508 college-aged gay males in Greater Boston has shown that about one-quarter have had anal intercourse without a condom in the last six months with a partner whose HIV status was unknown. The seroprevalence rates for these young men was 2.4 percent; however, among the young men who cannot or do not actually attend college, the rate was 9.4 percent (Mayer and Seage, 1994). This highlights the socioeconomic factors associated with increased risk for infection. In another survey of gay men ages eighteen to twenty-five in three medium-sized West Coast communities, 43 percent of those who were asked said they had had anal intercourse without a condom within the last six months (Hays et al., 1990). In Minnesota, a survey of young gay and bisexual adolescent males showed that 63 percent were either using injectable drugs or having unprotected anal intercourse (Remafedi, 1994).

The high prevalence of HIV in the gay community in general makes it more likely for a young gay man to become infected while exploring anal sex without a condom and experimenting with injectable drugs with his peers. In areas of some cities, like the Castro district in San Francisco and the Village in New York City, about half of the gay men are thought to be infected. Although it is difficult to be certain of the exact percentage of gay men who are already infected in cities like Boston and Pittsburgh, it is estimated that about one-quarter of the gay male population is HIV positive, with new infection occurring at an estimated annual rate of 2.6 percent (Mayer, 1995). At this rate of growth, it has been projected that the majority of twenty-year-old gay males will be infected with HIV in their lifetime (Hoover et al., 1991).

At one time, AIDS was considered by many youth to be an older man's disease, and they believed that if they were only sexual with their peers, they were not at risk. This belief was always erroneous, but now the levels of infection among young gay males are high enough to make this mistaken belief even more likely to result in infection, since the prevalence of HIV among adolescent gay males is so high.

These startling and tragic epidemiological trends forecast a huge and expanding AIDS epidemic among gay men. Lack of social support for gay youth increases the risk of infection as early as pre-adolescence, and the risk grows exponentially through adolescence and adulthood. With each passing year of the epidemic, it becomes increasingly difficult to envision a future for gay males that does not include HIV infection and ultimately AIDS. What, then, should be the goals of HIV prevention among gay youth? How do we make those goals realistic? And how do we achieve them?

THE GOALS OF HIV PREVENTION AMONG GAY YOUTH

Effective AIDS education for gay and bisexual youth is critically important for the future of the gay community and for the epidemiological course of the AIDS epidemic. The challenge for AIDS educators, therefore, is twofold: to provide education that limits the number of new infections among gay youth and simultaneously to prepare them for a long adult life during which they will successfully avoid infection. This is an element that is often lost in the discussions about adolescent AIDS education: Efforts targeting youth lay the groundwork for a lifelong goal of staying HIV negative. As has been mentioned, current projections estimate that the majority of twenty-year-old gay males will be infected with HIV or dead of AIDS by the time they are fifty; one-third will be infected by thirty years of age (Hoover et al., 1991). Many once believed that younger gay men would be spared the devastation of AIDS because they were to grow up into an established epidemic with its long-standing prevention education and changed community sexual norms. What we now realize is that educational efforts intended for adult gay men, while they undoubtedly saved scores of lives, have not succeeded in averting a second wave of AIDS in the gay community. In this context, the two goals of HIV prevention for young gay males—reducing the number of new infections during adolescence and preparing uninfected youth to remain HIV negative throughout adulthood—are intertwined.[2] But to meet these goals, it is necessary to have an accurate understanding of the prevention needs of gay adolescents.

UNDERSTANDING THE NEEDS OF GAY YOUTH

Young gay and bisexual males face a higher risk of becoming infected with HIV than most other young people. The immense physiological and psychological changes of adolescence, such as gaining independence from parents and family, defining and reconciling personal and social identities, the development of peer family relationships, and personal sexual experimentation, all may be complicated as one comes to understand that his sexual orientation is different from that of most of his peers and is not widely accepted in his culture. But because schools and other youth settings rarely recognize or acknowledge gay youth in their midst, resulting in precious few gay or gay-accepting adult role models and little peer support, gay youth usually lack opportunities to practice the social skills with members of the same gender which are crucial to their development. Therefore, they fail to establish authentic systems of peer, family, institutional, and social support for their emerging gay identities (Cranston, 1992; Odets, 1994).

Social discomfort and fear of homosexuality (especially homosexual activity among youth), the pervasive presumption that all adolescents are heterosexual, ignorance about the unique concerns and developmental issues of sexual minorities, and the failure of most adults to support gay youth in their psychological, social, and sexual development have severely limited the effectiveness of HIV prevention efforts for gay adolescents. Sadly, homophobia, heterosexism, and homoignorance have been the keystones of our nation's response to the AIDS epidemic from the beginning—with devastating effects to all gay people, and especially gay youth, who continue to be robbed of a crucial development task. By not being permitted to develop a positive sense of a homosexual self, gay youth often experience isolation from social systems that foster self-esteem and support a belief in one's ability and desire to avoid HIV infection.

The crucial challenge facing HIV prevention providers and health educators who work with gay youth is to promote positive feelings about being gay and a strong gay identity while we also provide accurate and age-appropriate information to gay youth who come from a variety of cultural and socioeconomic roots. The vexing question facing us is how to engage youth in a gay-positive culture of risk reduction that supports them in a desire to survive and increases their confidence in their ability to end the epidemic. In trying to answer that question, it is important to frame the risks facing gay youth in a way that avoids pathologizing adolescent homosexuality, but also does not trivialize the unique risks that gay youth face on a daily basis.

Gay youth are now commonly characterized as people who are two to three times more likely to commit suicide (Maguen, 1991); that they constitute a disproportionately larger percentage of urban street youth; that they are more likely to use and abuse substances, experience sexual exploitation or childhood sexual abuse; and have higher rates of STDs than their heterosexual peers (Paul et al., 1994; Stall, 1994). While gay youth may make up a larger proportion of the statistics for each of these risk factors, one must remember that any youth who has experienced serious trauma is much more likely to attempt and/or commit suicide, use substances, or isolate himself from mainstream society. It is also important to remember that while an estimated one-third of all gay male youth have attempted suicide, a full two-thirds have not. In fact, amidst primarily hostile social conditions, the vast majority of gay youth have been able to access an internal set of protective characteristics that have helped them remain safe against the odds.

The current and popular construction of gay adolescent homosexuality as a troubled condition has led us down a path of thinking that gay youth, as a result of their sexual orientation alone, are more likely to engage in risk-taking behaviors than anyone else. This has kept us from looking for, and then building upon, the characteristics of well-being that many gay youth clearly possess. In fact, the etiology of risk taking among gay youth is not their homosexuality, but rather the myriad other influences on their lives in combination with the social isolation that results from a culture unwilling to accept them as gay. Most gay youth overcome that isolation with little if any help from traditional peer, family, and professional networks; but many who lack those support systems will eventually succumb to HIV infection because they failed to develop a fundamental love of self that would lead them to view the whole of their lives as worthwhile.

A new and more positive view of adolescent homosexuality will lay a foundation for an expanded search for ways to help gay youth that goes beyond listing the numerous ways gay youth are at particularly high risk for a number of dangers. It would include seek-

ing out ways of fostering a strong and positive gay identity by building upon the uniquely strong and special traits that gay youth possess. It would also do something about the larger society that fails
to support, motivate, and empower gay youth in authentic and sex-
positive ways. By constructing adolescent homosexuality as pathological or somehow fundamentally disordered, we reject our
responsibility to accommodate the real needs of gay youth: to experience acceptance and equality in all aspects of social life and sexual
development and exploration, and to be acknowledged for the
strength of character that many of them possess.

RESPONDING TO THE NEEDS OF GAY YOUTH

Most gay young people are questioning their homosexual desires
throughout their teenage years and beyond; well into their twenties. As same-sex attractions emerge, gay youth often feel as if they
are the only ones to experience these feelings and, depending on
how negative the messages about homosexuality they received while
growing up, they are at greater risk for experiencing the kind of
internal turmoil that could result in self-destructive behaviors. Denial
is usually one way gay youth respond to their homosexual inclina-
tions; they may consider themselves to be going through a phase, or
they may go through a period of characterizing themselves as "bisexual." While true bisexuality exists as a sexual orientation, many
gay adolescents will choose this label as a safer transitional identity than homosexual. Another aspect of the denial may manifest
itself in a young person overcompensating for his initial suspicion
of homosexuality by becoming excessively heterosexually active.

As a rule, youth in early adolescence are not open about their
feelings to others, and fully expect to be rejected by their loved
ones. This fear of rejection is culturally constructed and is at the
root of the denial of emerging homosexuality that so many young
gay people experience. These factors—rejection and isolation—also
contribute to a negative image of one's self that directly influences
a gay person's ability and desire to consistently engage in life-affirming, healthy behaviors. A gay male who feels badly about himself and his homosexuality—and is pessimistic about his future
chances for happiness and fulfillment—is less likely to value his
life, believe in his ability to survive the epidemic, and consequently
use condoms when he engages in anal sex. Positive self-esteem is
the linchpin of one's ability to pursue healthy behavioral options.

Not to be excluded from this discussion is the young gay male
who has accepted his orientation, is sexually active, and might already be in a gay relationship in his mid- to late-teenage years or

early twenties. He is also at risk for HIV infection for some of the reasons mentioned previously and others. For him, condom use can symbolize distrust or lack of intimacy in a relationship, while the choice to have anal sex without a condom signifies a depth of commitment, trust, and love of his significant partner. While troubling, such behavior is completely understandable. Lovers want to know each other completely, and it can seem counterproductive to the evolution of a relationship to constantly have a physical barrier in place. In a recent survey of young gay men, 51 percent of the coupled respondents said they had unprotected anal sex to ejaculation over the previous two months (Hays et al., 1990). They felt as if their relationship was ready to withstand the consequences of that choice and they deeply desired to share this most intimate of acts with their special partner. While taking off the condom was viewed as a sign of trust and love, in many cases the partners were not absolutely certain of their HIV status.

In addition, many gay young men feel a sense of inevitability surrounding potential HIV infection. (This stands in sharp contrast to the often-referred-to sense of invincibility that is commonly identified as a cofactor for adolescent HIV risk-taking behaviors, as in Hays et al., 1990.) Some of these young people feel that it would be better to get infected with someone they love and trust to be there in the long run, rather than becoming infected by someone with whom there is no special relationship.

Australia's "Negotiated Safety" program engages couples in a decision-making process that might culminate in a couple's choice to engage in unprotected anal sex. By participating in a series of counseling sessions and facilitated discussions, and when both partners have gotten the results of HIV antibody tests, the men are faced with a decision whether to go ahead with anal sex without a condom. By acknowledging the fact that there is indeed a safe context for unprotected anal intercourse, young gay men can come to terms with the reality of AIDS without the demoralizing sex-negative overtones that mark many of the safe-sex messages currently used to educate youth. The intention of negotiated safety is to give a young gay male couple confidence in their ability to end the epidemic. But for this strategy to work, individuals must be able to engage in honest communication about emotionally volatile subjects, and the decision-making and maintenance regimens may be too demanding for most couples.

To address the complex psychological and social dynamics experienced by many gay youth, HIV and AIDS information needs to be presented within the context of the myriad concerns adolescents—and especially self-conscious, isolated, or sexually active gay ado-

lescents—are experiencing. Risk-taking behaviors and risk reduction take place within a broader context. The most at-risk gay adolescents are at risk precisely because they find the array of situations they
face too complex and confusing. Widespread violence and drug use;
unavailability of meaningful work or career paths; the health hazards of unreflective sexual experimentation; and the targeted violence, hatred, isolation, and ridicule they often experience, as well
as the confusing emotions associated with passionate and intense relationships, all contribute to an environment of risk that overwhelms a
young gay person's ability and, sometimes, desire to stay healthy.

SCHOOL-BASED HEALTH EDUCATION
FOR GAY ADOLESCENTS

AIDS and HIV are issues that should be addressed in comprehensive health education and contextualized in a discussion of continued health and well-being. In order for young people to address
their risks for HIV infection, they need to know how their bodies
work and have a broad understanding of personal health and
wellness, of related risk behaviors like substance use, and of human sexuality and STDs. Health education should be broad, and
continuously and incrementally delivered at all grade levels
(Cranston, 1992). As has been mentioned, self-esteem is the key to
self-efficacy and wellness, and promoting it for all students, including gay youth, should be the fundamental goal of comprehensive
health education.

AIDS education in the context of health education should accurately address the risk of male-to-male transmission while presenting homosexuality in a positive light. All too often, AIDS education
overemphasizes the risk of heterosexual transmission and barely
mentions the homosexual risk. It is hard to comprehend why this
may be the case, other than the fact that many AIDS and health
educators are either afraid of or prohibited from discussing homosexuality in frank terms. Schools can begin to correct this by including accurate and positive lessons on homosexuality in their
health curricula and by having gay speakers come to discuss homosexuality. As Cranston points out, schools often try to deflect some
of the homophobic responses that many adolescents accord HIV
prevention efforts by requesting that guest speakers who discuss
AIDS refrain from discussing homosexuality. This "has the unfortunate effect of eliminating one of the few educational situations in
which gay . . . issues can be discussed" (Cranston, 1992).

The most comprehensive school-based program should integrate
positive gay images into many other subject areas as well. This could

be done simply by acknowledging that countless literary, scientific, political, and historical figures were gay. A more daring program might try to explore some of the historical, social, and religious challenges faced by homosexuals over the generations, like the persecution of gays at various points in history, or the new evidence that some kind of same-sex bonding ritual was practiced in medieval Christianity, or the growing popularity of gay parenting. This kind of regular and sustained visibility in school curricula would not only help gay youth determine what kind of gay person they want to be, but would also confront and challenge the homophobia that drives many heterosexual youth to harm or threaten their gay peers.

In addition to building a fundamental love of self, gay youth also need to develop competency in a core set of skills that will help them make sound choices that preserve their well-being. Among these are communication skills that allow one to talk honestly and confidently about sex and sexual behaviors. Effective exercises that build communication skills increase the student's comfort level in talking about sex-related subjects, and could help him decide and effectively articulate his sexual desires and limits. Role-modeling exercises would help him develop necessary sexual negotiation and refusal skills.

Correct and accurate information, including how to use a condom, is the cornerstone of any health education curriculum, and educators cannot assume that gay students can generalize from information presented within the exclusive context of heterosexuality. Male-to-male anal intercourse and other homosexual behaviors should be explicitly and proactively discussed, since a gay student is unlikely to ask for specific information publicly, and is equally unlikely to extract relevant information from more generalized discussions.

COMMUNITY-BASED ACTIVITIES FOR HIV RISK REDUCTION

Keeping young gay males from becoming infected demands a comprehensive approach to promoting well-being, since the genesis of risk taking seems to come from the fundamental belief that there is no such thing as happy, healthy homosexuality. AIDS may seem, at best, just another of many reasons for a young gay male to live recklessly and only for the present. Because HIV is only one problem among many, AIDS educators need to deal in an holistic, integrated way with gay adolescents; they must address the entire range of issues, such as coming out, developing friendships and relationships, living arrangements, money and employment, and so on if they are to help gay youth achieve an empowered response to HIV.

This response includes, but goes beyond, school-based health education and must include the establishment of social outlets that are welcoming and affirming of gay youth. Social and recreational events can utilize peer leadership models to offer activities that encourage friendships and relationships with other gay or gay-affirming youth. Such programs could go a long way toward establishing a social norm that supports safer sexual behaviors and where the larger community places value on homosexuality and an HIV negative serostatus. This social approach to establishing new safer-sex norms and cultural values has already proven to be effective in reducing the rates of unprotected anal intercourse among men between the ages of eighteen and twenty-nine in Eugene, Oregon's "Mpowerment Project."

These kinds of projects are particularly appealing because they can attract large numbers of gay youth, thereby breaking through the isolation that many of them are known to experience. For example, a program in Boston called "Happy Times, Healthy Tomorrows," offered jointly by Boston Children's Services and Boston's Alliance of Gay and Lesbian Youth (BAGLY), expects 150 gay youth to attend a minimum of seventeen social events and includes a "street outreach" component that reaches an additional 200 to 600 gay adolescents. The goal of the program is to encourage positive social interactions that foster healthy emotional development in each person, thus leading to an increased desire to seek out life-affirming social interactions and relationships, and support for engaging in lower-risk sexual activities.

Recent research in Boston and San Francisco reveals that many gay and lesbian youth have little or no connection to a caring, supportive, adult gay community (Healthy Boston, 1995). This is a curious phenomenon, since it can be argued that the one positive outcome of the AIDS epidemic has been a stronger sense of gay community and gay community activism among adults. For a number of reasons, gay youth have yet to be fully integrated into that community experience. One reason for this has been the inability of many gay men and gay AIDS educators to extricate themselves from the internalized societal fear of intergenerational gay friendships.

Too often, gay adults are branded and stereotyped by heterosexuals and sometimes even by gay youth as pedophiles, promoters or recruiters for homosexuality, or people who would subvert the morality of youth (Smart, 1995). Gay men often shy away from supporting teens because they fear the stereotype or because they remember too well the pain of their own adolescence and prefer not to relive it by association with young people. What results from this complex dynamic is generational isolation, where "out" and visible adult gay role models are few and gay youth are not included in the many positive community-building institutions available to adult gay men. Therefore, education of the adult gay community is key to integrating gay youth in what could be protective gay community activities. In promoting communication and understanding between the adult and adolescent gay worlds, programs could try to capitalize on the enthusiasm of many out gay youth to do adult education and training on adolescent issues.

AIDS service organizations and other multiservice agencies have provided a venue for adult gay people to become engaged in and organized around the specific health concerns posed by AIDS. Interest in the gay AIDS epidemic on the part of government and the larger society has been minimal, because homosexuals are regarded by most to be a distasteful sexual minority; they have been consequently relegated to the ranks of other oppressed or marginalized groups on account of their sexual orientation. More out of dire necessity, perhaps, than for any other reason, the gay community itself has assessed and determined its own needs and designed its own effective models for education. In becoming critically engaged in educational events and activism projects, community members have gradually become personally and collectively empowered, motivated, and effective in doing something about ending AIDS. Gay men have taken control of their own sexual lives and developed a system of care that appropriately serves their needs. This community-empowerment approach—the so-called Freirian model, after the Brazilian educator Paulo Freire (Freire, 1970), which continues to be effective in reducing the number of new infections among adult gay men—unfortunately has not been widely duplicated for adolescents in general, nor for young sexual minorities. While the "empowerment" concept has been over-applied in certain settings, and sometimes wrongly or haphazardly implemented, it remains an approach that can lead to the development of a "community of conscience" among oppressed gay youth that gives them the perspective and resources they need to wrest control of their own sexual lives and work with adults to develop a network of services that meet their particular needs (Cranston, 1992). AIDS service organizations and youth-serving multiservice agencies are the most likely places for this approach to be attempted.

CONCLUSION

Many social institutions, like families, schools, and health and recreational centers are not willing to take on the issue of homosexuality in ways helpful to gay adolescents most likely to become infected with HIV. The political risks are considered too great, and it is often difficult for adults to come to consensus on how to best serve young gay people. Similarly, the gay community itself, for a variety of reasons, has not been explicitly involved with or supportive of gay youth, nor has it modeled for them the many positive ways gay people can live their lives in safety. A more comprehensive approach to reaching young gay males demands that schools, AIDS organizations, multiservice centers, and gay community institutions confront the homophobia that currently limits the effectiveness of prevention services. Adults must be willing to empower gay youth to take control of their sexual and relational lives; AIDS educators must insist on full integration of homosexuality into comprehensive health education curricula in schools; AIDS and multiservice organizations must strive to include gay youth in all aspects of education and activism; and adult gay men must accept the mantle of responsibility to serve as role models for gay youth. The foundation of any effort to reduce the risk of HIV infection among young gay males, however, is factual and positive information about homosexuality aggressively delivered; and an optimistic portrayal of gay life, culture, and sensibility. Stopping AIDS indeed starts with pride. The effort to provide all that needs to be done to protect the health of gay youth should be commensurate with the magnitude of the epidemic that awaits them if we fail.

NOTES

1. In this chapter, the terms *youth, adolescent,* and *adolescence* refer to individuals age eleven to twenty-four, and those sharing the developmental concerns of this age group who are somewhat older or younger.

2. One of the challenges of HIV prevention among any population is to determine what are the realistic goals of our efforts. Although our most desired outcome may be the elimination of all risks for infection and a complete and immediate halt to the spread of the epidemic, it is unreasonable to believe that this can be achieved in the absence of a medical vaccine. In fact, the overblown expectations of what we can accomplish in HIV prevention is often a barrier to finding support for experimental and innovative interventions. It also contributes to fatigue, discouragement, and burnout among prevention providers. Nevertheless, it is important not to set our goals too low, because we do know that HIV prevention efforts have saved countless and uncountable lives over the past fourteen years. The misconception that HIV prevention is failing is often rooted in unrealistic expectations for individual interventions and a desire for absolute solutions for the problem, such as the belief that condoms should be 100 percent effective before we recommend them as a method of risk reduction, or

the exclusive reliance on abstinence-based approaches to HIV prevention. One might suggest, as Jeff Stryker of the University of California at San Franciso Center for AIDS Prevention Studies did, that the very concept of HIV *prevention* is a misnomer. Perhaps it would be more accurate to speak of HIV *risk-reduction* efforts, whose goal is to *reduce the number of new HIV infections* to a level that will curb and eventually reverse the *epidemic* explosion of AIDS.

The now common "harm reduction" model of HIV education is increasingly the way prevention specialists refer to risk reduction. I try not to confuse the two terms and see them as fundamentally different. Harm reduction, which has its genesis in drug prevention, accepts that drug use is a harmful practice, but proposes an alternative to the all-or-nothing approach of twelve-step programs and the like. The principles of harm reduction attempt to mitigate the many harmful effects of drug use while not demanding abstinence from drug use; so, for example, in this model it is possible that a cocaine abuser could drink alcohol or use marijuana, if by doing so the harm of cocaine is avoided.

When talking about HIV prevention, infection is lethal, and there is no way to reduce the harm of that infection. Either you have HIV or you do not, and if you do, the harm of it cannot be mitigated. Furthermore, a notion that an intervention can positively influence the harmful effects of sexual intercourse seems to be fundamentally misguided, since sex is not, in and of itself, harmful. That model is simply sex negative and underestimates the positive and necessary role sexual activity and in particular sexual intercourse—whether it be vaginal or anal—plays in the lives of people. The goal of HIV education is to help the client assess when and with whom sexual intercourse may put him or her at risk for infection and motivate that client to avoid or reduce the risk of that situation. For this reason, risk reduction, and not harm reduction, seems to be the more appropriate conceptual framework for HIV education.

REFERENCES

Centers for Disease Control (CDC). (1995). HIV/AIDS Surveillance Summary as of May 1, 1995.

Cranston, K. (1992). HIV Education for Gay, Lesbian, and Bisexual Youth: Personal Risk, Personal Power, and the Community of Conscience. In *Coming Out of the Classroom Closet*, edited by Karen M. Harbeck. New York: Harrington Park Press.

Freire, P. (1970). *Pedagogy of the Oppressed.* New York: Seabury Press.

Hays, R. B., S. M. Kegeles, and T. J. Coates. (1990). High Risk Taking among Young Gay Men. *AIDS* 4: 901–907.

Healthy Boston Coalition Survey. (1995). Forthcoming.

Hoover, D. R., A. Munoz, V. Carey, et al. (1991). Estimating the 1978–1990 and Future Spread of Human Immunodeficiency Virus Type 1 in Subgroups of Homosexual Men. *American Journal of Epidemiology* 134: 1190–1205.

Lemp, G., G. Nieri, and the San Francisco Department of Public Health AIDS Office. (1994). Seroprevalence of HIV and Risk Behaviors among Young Homosexual and Bisexual Men: The San Francisco/Berkeley Young Men's Survey. *Journal of the American Medical Association* 272: 449–454.

Maguen, S. (1991). Teen Suicide: The Government's Cover-Up and America's Lost Children. *The Advocate*, 24 September.

Mayer, K. (1995). Epidemiology and Biological Factors. Presentation at the Summit on the Reduction of New HIV Infections among Gay Men in Massachusetts, 8–9 June, Boston.

Mayer, K., and G. Seage. (1994). HIV Seroprevalence among Gay College Men in Boston. Poster presented at the Tenth International Conference on AIDS, 7–12 August, Yokohama, Japan.

Odets, W. (1994). Psychosocial and Educational Challenges for the Gay and Bisexual Male Communities. Paper presented at the American Association of Physicians for Human Rights, AIDS Prevention Summit, 15–17 July, Dallas, Texas.

Paul, J., R. Stall, M. Crosby, et al. (1994). Correlates of Sexual Risk-Taking among Gay Male Substance Abusers. *Addiction* 89: 971–983.

Remafedi, G. (1991). Risk Factors for Attempted Suicide in Gay and Bisexual Youth. *Pediatrics* 87: 869–875.

Remafedi, G. (1994). Predictors of Unprotected Intercourse among Gay and Bisexual Youth: Knowledge, Beliefs and Behavior. *Pediatrics* 4: 901–907.

Rosenburg, P. S., R. J. Biggar, and J. J. Goedert. (1994). Declining Age at HIV Infection in the United States. *New England Journal of Medicine* 330: 789–790.

Sadownick, D. (1994). Untamed Youth. *Genre* (March): 37–43, 92.

Smart, G. (1995). Barriers to Effective AIDS Education for the Population of Gay Males between the Ages of 15 to 25. Paper presented at the Summit on the Reduction of New HIV Infections among Gay Men in Massachusetts, 8–9 June, Boston.

Stall, R. (1994). Intertwining Epidemics? A Short History of Research on the Relationship between Substance Use and the AIDS Epidemic among Gay Men. Paper presented at the Summit on HIV Prevention for Gay Men, Bisexuals, and Lesbians at Risk, Dallas, Texas.

Wendell, D., I. Onorato, D. Allen, E. McCray, and P. Sweeney. (1990). Seroprevalence among Adolescents and Young Adults in Selected Clinic Settings, United States, 1988–90. Paper presented at the Sixth International Conference on AIDS, San Francisco, California.

4

Targeting Education for Women Who Have Sex with Women

Mary K. Irvine

OVERVIEW

In the course of the HIV pandemic, lesbians and bisexual women have become the focus of a debate regarding sexual transmission and the demands made upon communities to uphold newer social norms for risk reduction. The years spent in debating their case have left these women close to where they started—with little data on how their practices relate to HIV and without strong modeling for the adoption of safer behaviors. There is one notable difference in their current position: The consequences of impaired risk assessment and of disaffection from prevention efforts are greater now than ever. The dearth of research about women with HIV and the particular silence on woman-to-woman transmission routes have fostered an attitude of skepticism and futility among women who have sex with women about the methods of safety proposed to them. These women find further cause for distrust in the changeable and contradictory nature of public statements about their risk.

Early in the epidemic, when "homosexuals" were established as the highest risk group for HIV/AIDS, lesbians and bisexual women found themselves categorically confused with gay and bisexual men in a familiar erasure of difference between groups not conforming to normative heterosexuality. Women in several countries could be rejected as blood donors if they claimed same-sex sexual activity on their donor screening forms (Richardson, 1994). The subgrouping of lesbians and bisexual women under a larger category of high-risk "homosexuals" seemed to represent a government priority of protecting the health of the mainstream white, noninjection drug–using, heterosexual population (the "innocent victims") by containing the virus in easily identified, socially undesirable populations. At this early stage of AIDS representations, social deviance served as a marker for risk (and guilt) of infection, while the "general population" was reassured by the popular and scientific media of its safety and blamelessness in the epidemic.

As AIDS knowledge and concepts of risk continued to develop, women having sex with women were epidemiologically relocated to a position of lesser risk in relation to the rest of the population. Lesbians, in particular, found themselves drawn right out of the picture of an epidemic in such defining instances as the Centers for Disease Control and Prevention (CDC) classification of them as women not having had sex with men since 1977, and the further description by a CDC spokesperson of lesbians as a group not having much sex at all (Stevens, 1993). The definition of this population by exclusion and the ranking of putatively discrete exposure categories have achieved a reassignment of lesbians to the category of lowest risk, and with it a justification of the neglect of women having sex with women in HIV/AIDS research and in funding of targeted programs for education and prevention. The official CDC confirmation of the nonrisk of lesbians has been echoed on more local levels by health professionals and even AIDS information hotlines (Stevens, 1993)—and has been desperately embraced as a promise of protection in the communities where women have sex with each other. At the same time that the CDC claims are routinely invoked as reason not to worry about HIV, the actual power of the CDC to recommend prevention strategies to lesbians and bisexual women has been jeopardized. An institution notorious for its desexualization of lesbian behaviors cannot expect to retain credibility when speaking to women who have sex with women about their possible risks for HIV or other STDs.

Among the diverse communities redefined in relation to the pandemic, lesbians and bisexual women represent a peculiar position of conflict between HIV prevention messages received and sexual practices widely accepted and continued without revision. On the one hand, lesbians and bisexual women have been inundated with general information about HIV/AIDS and the importance of adopting safer-sex practices as a new community standard. For some HIV educators and activists, lesbians and bisexual women have merited attention as a group that might readily be targeted through means already tested with gay and bisexual male communities (Patton, 1991). The relatively recent formation of political coalitions between gay, lesbian, and bisexual people has sparked hopes that these groups would together find a way to eliminate public ignorance about their numbers, identities, and concerns and to stop the spread of HIV/AIDS in their communities.

On the other hand, women who have sex with women have been left to make choices about their sexual health without the benefit of HIV/AIDS research addressing woman-to-woman routes of viral transmission, female (especially early) symptomatology of the illness, or secure methods of preventing transmission between women. Their coalitions with gay and bisexual male AIDS activists have often broken down over issues of class, race, and gender—issues arising, in part, from the disproportionately high rates of female infections among working-class women and women of color. Lesbian and bisexual women have been accused of "virus envy" (Richardson, 1994:159) when beginning to organize around HIV issues in their own communities, rather than functioning in a purely deferential, supportive, and sympathetic role with respect to recognized communities at risk. In this environment of isolation and of competing desires for the truth and for a disengagement from the fray of the epidemic, women who have sex with women make their decisions about risk taking and behavioral change.

WOMEN AT RISK

A community HIV prevention and participatory research project conducted by Lyon-Martin Women's Health Services Clinic in San Francisco set, as its primary goal, the defeat of a "cultural construction of immunity" pervasive in the population of women having sex with women (Stevens and Hall, 1994a:8). This chapter uses the reports on the first and second years (1993 and 1994) of the Lyon-Martin project, along with other report materials dealing with the San Francisco Bay Area population of women who have sex with women, in order to demonstrate patterns of risk behavior common to many of these women imagined outside of the realm of HIV transmission. Perhaps even more distressing than these behaviors are the accompanying patterns of denial and of radically contingent and contradictory personal assessments of risk and safety, which appear in the reports as the dominant context for sex between women

in these communities. The few investigations made into the negotiation of safer practices by women having sex with women reveal
their decisions to be both culturally overdetermined and individually rationalized. In their attempts to fit themselves into a larger
picture of the epidemic, these women find themselves unable to
trust the general media and unwilling to make great personal sacri-
fices until they have a weightier, more scientific reason for them
than their private doubts. The health-related decision making performed by lesbians and bisexual women in an atmosphere of denial
and disorientation may also provide insight into elements of the
decision making that occurs in those communities classified as
higher risk (e.g., the responses of gay and bisexual male communities to the constantly shifting official stance on risk from perform-
ing fellatio, and particularly from swallowing pre-ejaculatory fluid).

The fairly recent behavioral studies that have collected data on
women having sex with women indicate that they engage in risky
activities at an alarming rate, even if no consideration is given to
unprotected sex with other women as a potential risk. A study by
Project AWARE (the Association for Women's AIDS Research and
Education) selected its sample of 711 Bay Area women for (1) involvement with a high-risk male sexual partner in the past three
years or (2) involvement with ten or more sexual partners of any
gender during the same three-year period. What it found in its participants—recruited through outreach into neighborhoods with high
rates of poverty, crime, and drug use—was an unexpectedly large
number of women who reported at least one female sexual partner
during the past three years (329, or 41%), and a correlation between
the history of female sexual partners and higher-risk behaviors. The
women reporting at least one female sexual partner in the past three
years more frequently reported injection drug use (76%) than women
without female sexual partners (42%). They were also twice as likely
to report anal sex with a male partner (33% versus 16%) than women
with no female sexual partners. In this study, only 24 percent of the
women described themselves as lesbian or bisexual. While those
who reported sex with at least one woman did not significantly
differ in their rate of HIV infection from those who did not report
this behavior (10% versus 11%), the women who self-identified as
lesbian or bisexual showed higher rates of infection (14%) than those
who did not so identify (Cohen, 1993). These data suggest that, although behavior and identity are not mutually defining, a socially
marginal identity in certain environments may increase the likelihood or the frequency of higher-risk behaviors.

Cohen cites the National AIDS Demonstration Research Project
(NADR) data on HIV risk among injection drug users and their sexual

partners, because those data do indicate a higher rate of seroconversion among women who reported any same-sex partners than among those who did not. The NADR data also reveal that these women were more frequently sharing syringes and having survival or commercial sex (Cohen, 1993). While neither of these studies specifically set out to gather information on the population of women having sex with women, both generated data on this population to suggest its potential as a separate study group. Together, these studies illustrate the public-health pitfalls which accompany a wedding of identity to behavior and an assurance of low risk. The particularly high level of HIV infection among lesbian and bisexual participants in the AWARE study, which recruited from inner-city street locations and had a largely black sample (69%), underscores the importance of examining how race and class interact with risk factors and cofactors affecting the population of women who have sex with women.

Looking at the steady rise in HIV seroconversions among women in general (female infections are increasing at about four times the rate of male infections), we can begin to imagine the significance that these figures may have for the movement of HIV in this subgroup of the population of women. In the San Francisco Department of Public Health (SFDPH) AIDS Office "HIV Seroprevalence Report," which now includes "Lesbian/Bisexual" as a distinct transmission category for women, it is still difficult to evaluate the prevalence of HIV locally among lesbians and bisexual women, because of the exclusion of current or former (since 1978) injection drug users from their category (SFDPH, 1995b). Generally speaking, it is less feasible to collect HIV seroprevalence data than it is to determine AIDS prevalence in a population. In a population group which is still experiencing the early stages of its own epidemic, it is likely that the increasing rates of HIV transmission will not become obvious from AIDS prevalence figures for some years. More important, lesbians and bisexual women are still less likely than members of other populations at risk to get tested or to be checked by a clinician for signs of HIV infection, because of the myth of their immunity. As a result, HIV positive women in this community are commonly not diagnosed or counted in surveillance data until they have become ill with AIDS.

In a 1993 study conducted by the SFDPH, Berkeley Department of Health and Human Services, and the Division of HIV/AIDS of the CDC, the rate of HIV in a group of 498 lesbian and bisexual women sampled at twenty-five Berkeley and San Francisco locations was more than three times as high as that estimated for all adult and adolescent women in San Francisco (SFDPH Surveillance, 1993).

This suggests that the assignment of lesbians and bisexual women to a position of minimal risk in the epidemic is not only misleading, but may have entrenched risk-taking behaviors which have boosted the rates of transmission in this population. While this and the handful of other studies conducted on the population of women who have sex with women provide information admittedly limited by smaller sample size, they manage to point up the failure of "risk groups" and their association with discrete identities to account for the actual sexual and drug-related practices circulating within and among diverse communities and continuing to put people at risk for HIV.

THE LYON-MARTIN SAN FRANCISCO PROJECT

The AmFAR Targeted Education Grant to Lyon-Martin Women's Health Services, "HIV Risk Reduction for Three Subgroups of Lesbian and Bisexual Women in San Francisco," began with the hope of reaching lesbians and bisexual women considering pregnancy; lesbian and bisexual partners of HIV positive women; and lesbians and bisexual women attending women's bars, dance clubs, and sex clubs (Stevens, 1993). The first part of the grant did not succeed in meeting its goals for education of potentially parenting lesbians at risk for HIV, largely because the women who used the service tended already to be well educated about HIV and were more interested in finding out about other kinds of concerns and resources around lesbian and bisexual parenting. In both years that this part of the grant was operating, women attending the parenting seminars or calling the hotline overrepresented Euro-American, well-educated, well-employed, higher-income women (Stevens, 1993; Stevens and Hall, 1994a, 1994b). Stevens summarizes as follows: "As the peer educator who was responsible for operating the parenting hotline suggested, it may be community outreach efforts rather than services provided at the clinic that hold the most promise for contacting diverse segments of the lesbian and bisexual women's community who are getting pregnant and are at risk for contracting HIV" (Stevens and Hall, 1994b:2). Part two of the grant also missed its mark for inclusion and numbers of women attending group or individual counseling sessions and couples retreats, apparently because of an informally developed policy requiring participants to be clean and sober. Project staff decided that another, separate structure would have to be developed to address issues of ongoing drug and alcohol use alongside issues of involvement with an HIV positive partner. The evaluation points out that the women likely to be in greatest need of support for dealing with mixed-serostatus ("discordant" or "magnetic") relationships with other women were those still using substances (Stevens and Hall, 1994a).

The most successful part of the Lyon-Martin/AmFAR grant project was the segment targeting young women attending women's bars, dance clubs, sex clubs, and—in year two—community events. This part of the grant carried out research on the population's risk-taking behaviors and their motivating factors, while providing context-specific HIV education and prevention tailored to strengthen areas of knowledge shown lacking or confused in individual women during one-on-one interviews (Stevens, 1993). This dually focused project enacted participatory research in a population which had been overlooked both in data collection and in peer modeling and education around sexual health and safety issues.

The evaluation of this project documents the ways in which the carefully selected and trained team of educators (identified on their outreach T-shirts as "The Safer Sex Sluts") approached their goal of promoting behavioral change on the levels of individual decision making, relational and interpersonal negotiations of sexual encounters, and cultural environment. The team implemented an intervention characterized by four elements: "a combined group and individual approach, continuity over time, cultural competence, and context-specific education" (Stevens and Hall, 1994b:18). This Lyon-Martin project seems effectively and inclusively to have encouraged knowledge-enhancement and behavioral change in its target population; and in the process it managed to record a total of 1,189 separate interviews treating the HIV-related knowledge, attitudes, beliefs, and behaviors of self-identified lesbians and bisexual women in San Francisco. For these two reasons, this chapter will frequently refer to its findings for their illustration of roadblocks to the adoption of safer-sex practices by women having sex with women and of viable approaches to moving beyond these obstacles.

WAITING FOR EVIDENCE: RESPONSES TO GAPS IN RESEARCH ON WOMAN-TO-WOMAN TRANSMISSION

A recurrent theme in the "partners" and the "nightspots/community events" portions of the Lyon-Martin project was the frustration of lesbians and bisexual women at not being able to access reliable or specific information about the transmission of HIV through woman–woman sexual activities. As a result of the epidemiological and public-informational inattention to the varieties of woman–woman sexual behaviors and of female body fluids and membranes, women in this population find themselves pressed to make health- and life-affecting decisions based on very little information. In the

SFDPH AIDS Office report on a community-based health survey of 483 San Francisco lesbians and bisexual women, 99.6 percent of respondents reported having been exposed to some HIV prevention message in the past year—50 percent of these recalled messages about safe sex in general, 43 percent recalled promotions of condom use, 20 percent recalled the message that everyone is at risk, 14 percent recalled information about needle-cleaning or not sharing needles, and 10 percent recalled HIV testing promotion. When asked about HIV prevention messages specifically dealing with sex between women, 62 percent reported having been exposed to messages of this kind—51 percent of these recalled the promotion of specific safer-sex activities, 23 percent recalled the message that lesbians are at risk, and 22 percent recalled the message that women are at risk (SFDPH Prevention, 1993).

These statistics suggest that women who have sex with women in the San Francisco area are by no means unaware of the general informational efforts toward HIV prevention, but that only a slight majority have been exposed to HIV prevention messages targeting their population. Of the messages received about women having sex with women, nearly one-half focused on the assertion of presence of risk, leaving just about one-half which actually mentioned specific measures for prevention. This leaves us with over two-thirds of the total sample who did not report having seen or heard messages about the actual practice of safer-sex activities between women. It is unsurprising, then, that many of the women interviewed by the Lyon-Martin team expressed insecurities about the practical application of safer-sex standards and cited this awkwardness and confusion as the reason they had not been engaging in safer sex (Stevens, 1993). The majority of women interviewed during the first year of the intervention indicated that they were hearing about woman-to-woman HIV prevention for the first time through the Lyon-Martin project (Stevens, 1993).

The relatively low circulation of specific information about the practice of safer sex between women has bolstered the communal construction of immunity, in that women are likely to infer that they have not been targeted with this kind of information for the simple reason that they are not expected to take seriously or literally the message that "everyone is at risk." Even faced with more recent evidence or direct personal experience demonstrating the existence of HIV/AIDS among lesbians and bisexual women, members of these communities continue to dismiss the possibility of their own risk, assuming that the HIV positive women they know or hear about contracted the virus through sex with men or injection drug use.[1] In obedience to the notion of "risk groups," which formed the terms and structure of HIV/AIDS discourse from the beginning of the epidemic, women having sex with women have often employed, as their only method of risk reduction, a kind of intuition-based, spoken history–based, or sexual identity–based "weeding out" of risk-associated women from what have become conveniently imagined as the margins of the lesbian and bisexual community. At these projected pollutive fringes, women too old, too young, too close to men, too promiscuous with women, too S/M, too vanilla, too honest, too secretive, too druggy, and so forth for sex without risk threaten to work their way in among the "real" lesbians who have nothing to hide or tell about HIV. The method of risk reduction by exclusion of such women quickly shows its seams; most women in the community become ineligible as lovers when these criteria are applied. Once a woman begins to feel attracted or close to another woman sexually, though, the possibility that her chosen partner might be one of these menaces to the integrity of the community is most often discarded and safe sex presumed unnecessary. An overly rigid and simplistic standard of proper lesbian conduct becomes subject to doubt in the face of living, breathing women and their desires, but there has not yet risen another standard that could gain the loyalty and currency needed to replace it.

In their necessarily ungrounded and individualized decision making about sexual risk-taking, lesbians and bisexual women sometimes resort to a kind of cart-before-the-horse logic: "I am very careful before I trust another person. So if it comes to the point of having sex with that person, she must be trustworthy" (Stevens, 1993:13) or, "I've never had any diseases and no lover of mine would have anything either" (Stevens, 1993:11). In both of these claims, risk is clearly removed from a context of individual behaviors that could be changed in the interests of safety, and is collapsed with a loosely understood but supposedly self-evident untrustworthy or morally deficient character. The idea that people of this character, and with them risk, can be avoided through the normal operations of a woman's instincts or feelings furthers the essentialization of lesbians as naturally protected from risk.

COMMON RISK BEHAVIORS

The actual behaviors reported by self-described lesbians frequently reveal themselves to be at odds with the lesbian identity idealized by epidemiologists and by women partnering with women. Not only do many lesbians consensually have sex with men even after "coming out," but they are often less prepared than heterosexual or bisexual women to use condoms or to employ other methods of safety with men (Stevens and Hall, 1994a). Risk taking with men can be influenced by a number of behaviors and attitudes accompanying those encounters. Reports of these include a use of substances increasing the chances of being sexual with a partner who would not usually be considered, a lack of planning for sex with men (no matter how often it may occur) because it does not fit one's self-definition, a practice of survival sex where money or drugs are at stake, and an unpreparedness to argue or engage with men about condoms (Stevens, 1993). For some women accustomed to sex with other women, an atmosphere of the "carnivalesque" surrounding sex with men may support unsafe behaviors, which can be viewed as existing in a kind of alternate universe. It is also important to acknowledge the participation of many lesbians and bisexual women in the sex industry, which can limit their choices around safety and encourage risk taking in exchange for economic benefit.

Lesbian and bisexual injection drug users have also reported sharing needles with each other, under the assumption that it would be safe to shoot with other women like themselves (Stevens, 1993). Patton describes a 1992 study providing statistical evidence for "significant women-only drug injection groups" (Patton, 1994:74). While injection drug use has been jettisoned from the community self-imaging of lesbians, its practice among women who have sex with women seems fairly consistent with the modalities of other, more accepted "lesbian" behaviors.

All three reports focusing on the risk behaviors of San Francisco Bay Area lesbian and bisexual women indicate high rates of sex, often unprotected, with gay and bisexual men. In the San Francisco/Berkeley Women's Survey, 14.6 percent of the sample of lesbian and bisexual women reported unprotected oral sex with gay or bisexual men, 9.6 percent unprotected vaginal sex, and 3.2 percent unprotected anal sex (SFDPH Surveillance, 1993). Of the total sample, 11 percent of the SFDPH Prevention branch study reported sex (not specified as protected or unprotected) with gay or bisexual men in the past three years (SFDPH Prevention, 1993). The Lyon-Martin interviews provided personal testimony to the prevalence of sex with gay and bisexual men among lesbians and bisexual women, who sometimes went unprotected in the spirit of experimentation (Stevens and Hall, 1994a). The construction of cultural immunity seems able to cut across all areas of risk to women who have sex with women. Having been consolidated under the sign of safety due to lack of information and research, much of the lesbian and bisexual female population is still scrambling to hold its place under that sign, despite the emergence of evidence contradicting its validity.

Women who have sex with other women do so in a crossfire of opposing messages about their relation to the HIV/AIDS epidemic. It is in attempting to strike a balance between, for example, the safer-sex slogan widely promoted in the larger gay and bisexual community, "100% safe 100% of the time," and the perseverant classification of lesbians and bisexual women as a "low-risk" group, that women sleeping with women tend to suffer from loss of perspective and from discontinuities in their sexual negotiations. In the first year of the Lyon-Martin project, voluntarily reported risk behaviors among the lesbian and bisexual women interviewed included the following: (1) injection drug use, 6 percent—likely underreported, due to the stigma attached to this practice in the community; (2) regular unprotected sex with women, 75 percent; (3) regular unprotected sex with men, 15 percent; and (4) inconsistent practice of safer sex with men and women, 25 percent (Stevens, 1993). The 1993 SFDPH report found that 70 percent of lesbian and bisexual women surveyed agreed with the statement, "Many of my friends have unsafe sex" (SFDPH Prevention, 1993:26). While 87 percent also agreed with the statement, "AIDS has greatly impacted me personally" (SFDPH Prevention, 1993:26), few of the 483 respondents felt that women having sex with women have changed their behaviors because of HIV/AIDS or tried to protect themselves against STDs in encounters with other women. Apparently, the HIV-educational imperative that everyone form a single, firm policy of safety is either missing the population of women who have sex with women or is reaching it in unintentional and uncontrolled ways.

ONCE-REMOVED RELATIONSHIPS TO HIV
AND THE BREAKDOWN OF SELF-CARE

One explanation for the apparent discrepancy between the statements with which SFDPH survey participants aligned themselves is that most women in this population do feel greatly impacted by the epidemic, but generally feel it in connection to others whom they know to be at risk or seropositive for HIV, rather than feeling an impact on their own social circles and sexual practices. Their concern for sexual safety seems often to reflect a concern for the safety of a larger gay/lesbian/bisexual community and a sense of solidarity with other groups fighting their own battles against HIV. The relation of lesbians and bisexual women to the HIV/AIDS epidemic can be described as colored by a communal experience of "survivor guilt," which is supported by constitutions of the lesbian and bisexual women's population as exceptional in its nonrisk status. Survivor guilt affecting individual lesbian and bisexual partners of HIV positive women was recognized in the Lyon-Martin research project as contributing to unprotected sexual encounters and other self-endangering behaviors (Stevens, 1993). When made so constantly aware of the serious and immediate problems of their HIV positive loved ones, it proved difficult for these HIV negative women to maintain their strategies for self-care. In a similar manner, the experience of many lesbian and bisexual women of a more diffuse, community-level survivor guilt may compound their difficulties with acknowledging HIV as a personally relevant health issue and responding with consistent, reliable methods of risk reduction.

EQUALITY AND DIFFERENCE IN HIV EDUCATION

At many points during the past fifteen years, groups of lesbians and bisexual women have felt their personal, social, political, economic, or health-related concerns overlapping with those of gay and bisexual men organizing themselves around HIV/AIDS issues. At the same time, HIV prevention efforts beginning to address women who have sex with women have set as a goal for women's educational projects, messages, and materials an eventual equivalency with the projects, messages, and materials targeted to gay and bisexual men. Beyond striving after an equal level of visibility, the designers of HIV education and prevention for lesbians and bisexual women have frequently attempted a cut-and-paste style of directly adopting messages, safer-sex tools, slogans, images, and favored media and educational strategies from popular gay and bisexual men's programs. In this manner, equal or comparable status and success have been sought at the expense of difference or a recognition of the altering contexts of these representations when presented to women, and specifically to the women partnering with other women who are most at risk for HIV—women whose racial, ethnic, and income groups are disconnected from the most visible and established pockets of the gay community. As a result of the race for equal time and parallel education, many women who have sex with women continue to buy T-shirts with catchy slogans and glamorous representations of lesbian safer sex, to note appreciatively or even pick up the dental dams offered them at health fairs and community events or clinics, to wear prevention message buttons at the annual Lesbian/Gay/Bisexual/Transgender Pride Parade, to make and to watch women's safer-sex videos and presentations, and otherwise to pay allegiance to the community standard of sexual safety—perhaps out of a general desire to see themselves and their desires made visible and intelligible in public forums, or out of an understanding that they cannot take for granted any amount of inclusion of lesbians and bisexual women in HIV/AIDS or other public-health discourses. Through all this, though, their personal sexual practices appear for the most part to consist of much less determinate and less coherent convictions about active risk aversion.

Especially for members of a group repeatedly told that the chances of viral transmission in their sexual exchanges are negligible, the rigidity of a "no exceptions" model for prevention measures is difficult to accept and maintain. When the endorsements of safer sex in the lesbian and bisexual community find themselves unmatched by women's behaviors, the sense of a continuum of risk and safety tends to be lost to a sense of failure to live up to the requirements of safer sex. By hastily extending these models of safety—without regard for their performance as incredible, unattainable, and ultimately alienating prescriptions for the newly targeted population—HIV education efforts threaten to widen the gap between the public and political face of lesbian and bisexual women's sexual standards and the more private and individualized practices of sex, to the point of a complete disassociation of the two. It is not just women having sex with women who stand to lose from the stubborn adherence to models of risk reduction developed for a generalized, white gay and bisexual male population; education targeting other populations will never benefit from the experience of lesbians and bisexual women if it does not allow for the possibility of a productive shift in its underlying assumptions about the ways people learn, communicate, and make decisions about sexual practices—not to mention the ways they have sex.

SACRED OBJECTS OF EDUCATION: THE DENTAL DAM

The dental dam holds a special place in safer-sex promotions for lesbians and bisexual women as the most obviously unconvincing attempt at parallelism to gay and bisexual men's condom promotions. Designed for oral surgery and unmodified for the purposes of oral sex, the dam has not yet been displaced as the focus of educational representations of safer sex between women.[2] The use of this thick, small, often artificially flavored (for kids who dread going to the dentist, not for sex) and corn starch–dusted square of latex was prescribed for woman-to-woman oral sex before any specific or reliable information about women's vaginal fluids and membranes could be gleaned from existing HIV/AIDS research. Many women have evinced a reasonable amount of suspicion about this order that they "use latex now, ask questions later," and about the particular choice of the dental dam as fitted to the needs of women having sex with women. For many, the dam has come to represent the insensitivity of HIV/AIDS "experts" and educators to the realities of female sexual exchanges. Its promoters have been charged with denying the possibility of female ejaculation, imagining that women having sex do not need their hands free for anything but the task of holding a tiny square in place, assuming that women do not move around or cover much erogenous territory during oral sex, and failing to see the importance to women of the kind of sensation that does not penetrate a barrier as thick and unwieldy as the dam. For any number of reasons, the dental dam has failed to attain popularity among the lesbians and bisexual women to whom it was so enthusiastically promoted in an attempt to identify a safer-sex tool and practice "just for women." The use of plastic wrap and of cut and uncut condoms and gloves have all seemed to hold more promise as safer-sex tools for this population, but these carry their own safety hazards, negative or nonerotic associations, and disappointments.

In the Lyon-Martin project, women participating in the one-on-one interviews and women attending the meetings and retreats for members of HIV positive/negative couples agreed in their assessment of oral–genital sexual contact between women as the hardest activity to adapt to safer-sex standards (Stevens and Hall, 1994b). However, the dental dam has been the constant and often the limit of woman-to-woman representation in safer-sex campaigns. Ironically, cunnilingus is at one and the same time the act that has been aggressively targeted for behavioral change in this population, the act defining woman-to-woman sexuality in the public mind, and the act widely associated with the peculiarly low risk of lesbians and bisexual women in the first place. Vaginal and anal penetration (such as fisting), cutting and blood play, and the sharing of sex toys have largely been ignored as potential transmission routes between women and as behaviors to be targeted for risk reduction.

A number of the women who were contacted through the Lyon-Martin project expressed that oral–genital sex constitutes the quintessential element of lesbian sexuality. As one woman summarized, "It is like heterosexuals having intercourse. If I haven't done it, I feel like I haven't had sex at all" (Stevens and Hall, 1994b:5). Stevens notes that statements like this indicate the linkage of certain sexual activities with constructions of lesbian identity, and that a protective attitude toward the unmediated practice of oral sex on women may represent a larger concern about safer-sex practices rupturing the meaningful core of lesbian existence. In observing this point of resistance to safer-sex practices, Stevens wonders if other forms of sexual expression between women might achieve this kind of liberatory, identity-forming, and intimacy-oriented status. She questions whether the centering of oral–genital contact may derive from a "socialization into women-to-women sexual practices," and whether there might be cultural or age-related variances in the ways that such practices are felt and understood (Stevens and Hall, 1994b:6). It seems that the attempt to encapsulate lesbian sexuality (safer or not) in the image of oral–genital contact might be questioned as a developmental view of "real" lesbian sexual relations, and might be challenged by the reclaiming among many out lesbian, gay, bisexual, and transgendered people of a "polymorphous perversity," or a proliferation of nontraditional sexual expressions. While women who feel identified with the act of oral sex with women may be more inclined to react to safer-sex messages with unease about their regulatory and prescriptive values, these women might also be expected to recognize the subtler manipulations at work in the insistence on oral–genital sex as the consummation of woman-to-woman sexuality.

A final question that might be asked about the guarded status of oral sex between women as a site of identity constitution is whether existing representations of safety in woman-to-woman sexual encounters have overly depended upon and stabilized the concept of this singular sexual practice as defining of lesbian and bisexual women's erotic existence. The exclusive focus on latex barriers for oral sex between women, like the focus on the condom as the sign of safety between men or between men and women, privileges the act being modified for safety as the essential act (cunnilingus, anal intercourse, and vaginal intercourse, respectively) of the sexual subgroup in question. A genuine plurality of safer-sex representations would seem more appropriate to the needs of populations whose erotic behaviors cannot be viewed as always driving toward a single act, and who are being asked to change their customary behaviors for the purpose of risk reduction.

The practical difficulties women described having with safer techniques for oral sex included the inadequacy of barriers available, the incompatibility of barrier use with the multisensory pleasures of oral–genital contact, the inhibitory function of latex for intimacy, and the lack of evidence demonstrating either the necessity of this precaution or its effectiveness in preventing HIV transmission between women. As Stevens summarizes, "The general notion expressed in these interviews was that existing latex barriers are not easily adaptable for use by women and are geared more for use by men" (Stevens and Hall, 1994b:15). One woman suggested that the kinds of barriers that could be developed to serve more of the needs of women who have sex with women would also be important to straight women for safer sex with men (Stevens and Hall, 1994b).

Lodged in this translation between target populations is a problem with the promotion of the dental dam, larger even than its physical and erotic deficiencies: There appears to have been little or no expectation that anyone but lesbians and bisexual women would ever use the dental dam. It was offered up almost exclusively to the population of women who have sex with women in a simplistic attempt to find *something* for these women to do with each other in the way of HIV risk reduction. So that nobody should feel "left out" of safer-sex education, lesbians and bisexual women were encouraged to use dental dams with each other, while heterosexual women and men were never informed about dams, presumably because they already had condoms.

MIXED EDUCATIONAL MESSAGES: THE SELECTIVE RECOGNITION OF RISK

The targeting of only lesbians and bisexual women with instruction in the uses of barriers for oral–genital contact with women suggests itself as a purely symbolic gesture. Logically, if educators believed that this kind of contact constituted a risk, then heterosexual men might be expected to use them as well. This elision in HIV educational constructs of oral–genital contact with women as a risk to men lends itself to a number of unintended interpretations: that there is something peculiarly "wrong" and "sickening" about women having oral sex with each other, that men do not practice oral sex on women, that dental dams are just about lesbians and bisexual women becoming visible and not about anyone's practice, or that safer sex is being deployed as part of a larger agenda for the regulation and containment of nontraditional and female sexual expressions. If health educators expect to build trust and to reach women having sex with women, then this kind of inconsistency in the information distributed to targeted populations must be eliminated, and more studies must be performed on the presence of HIV in particular fluids (menstrual blood, vaginal or cervical secretions, female ejaculate, yeast or gardnerella-heavy vaginal fluids, and so forth) that can be passed from women to their partners, regardless of gender.[3]

SEX BEYOND COMMUNITY: LIVING THROUGH THE MAINSTREAM

Significant progress in HIV education might be made through the recognition that, as educational campaigns directed toward lesbians and bisexual women are fairly small, local, and recent, the more mainstream informational campaigns addressing a presumed-heterosexual audience may often form the basis of HIV knowledge for women having sex with women. Those women who have sex with women but do not receive much HIV information specifically addressing their sexual activities will commonly make inferences to their own practices from generally distributed safety messages. Women who are more difficult to target as members of a consolidated lesbian and bisexual community—because of closetedness, geographic isolation, or social or sexual nonidentity with such a community—would be particularly ill-served by the split between mainstream HIV educational messages and lesbian and bisexual HIV educational messages.

The Lyon-Martin and two SFDPH reports on health behaviors of lesbians and bisexual women in the Bay Area all specify that their samples can only be expected to represent the population in their geographic location of *socially active* women who have sex with women. It would seem that a very different strategy for sampling and then for targeting information would have to be attempted in order to research, and to reach with educational messages, the women who have sex with other women outside of a supportive community context. It may be that inclusion in mainstream educational campaigns (and campaigns targeting communities of color, substance users, or sex workers) of the mention of sexual activities between women would encourage the reception of valuable risk-reduction information without its strict attachment to preconceived identity groups or subcultures. More generally speaking, the reorganization of HIV prevention projects according to the range of sexual and drug-related behaviors possible in a target group for transmission of HIV, and a simultaneous de-emphasis of identity-based images of transmission, might manage to pick up where previous strategies of education seem to have left off—by reaching those whose risks for HIV go unrecognized or "unspecified" in epidemiological accounts.

SOMETIMES SOMEWHAT SAFE: LET'S BE MONOGAMOUS TONIGHT

Instead of a communal norm of sexual safety as "100%, 100% of the time," what the Lyon-Martin study witnessed among lesbians and bisexual women attempting safer sex was a tendency toward an inconsistent and contextually dependent practice of risk-reduction techniques. The women interviewed stipulated conditions for the practice of safer sex that sometimes cancelled each other; some could imagine becoming comfortable with the techniques of safer sex only with a primary partner who would understand, encourage, and support them in changing their behaviors. Others expressed a complete inability to imagine integrating these techniques into an established, serious sexual relationship, where suggesting safer sex might threaten the trust between partners, or where unsafe sex was considered the "perk" of being in a steady relationship.

The Lyon-Martin study found that monogamy was most commonly considered the ideal form of risk reduction. However, the definitions of monogamy ranged from the traditional sense of a long-term and exclusive relationship to any sexual relationship that one might get into: "I'm monogamous with whomever I'm with" (Stevens, 1993:13). While the loose situating of monogamy as a place for acceptable risk taking would suggest that encounters considered to be casual would then more readily agree with safer-sex techniques, the level of general discomfort and unfamiliarity with safer sex among the sample of women sometimes made it too hard to do or too loaded an issue to confront with strangers: "Safer sex is too intimate a conversation for a one night stand" (Stevens and Hall, 1994a:14). To some of the women interviewed, safer-sex techniques were much easier to demand with men (who were more used to addressing concerns about pregnancy and STDs) than with other women. However, other women described the kinds of responses they had gotten from men about condoms as "mean" and intimidating (Stevens and Hall, 1994a:14), while the women with whom they had sex appeared to be more generally sensitive and approachable. In each of these situations, the dominant theme was that many women having sex with women would not be able to integrate safer-sex practices into their experience of sex unless their partners either initiated preventive techniques or immediately responded well to suggestions of their use. Many lesbians and bisexual women seemed to believe that making a policy of safer sex would require them to become undesirably assertive and forceful.

Some women had conceded certain sexual practices identified as risky, but had reached their limit of tolerance for risk reduction with those concessions and so were still putting themselves at risk with other behaviors. A similar approach, discussed earlier in this chapter, was the omission of certain "types" of people (generally based on identity and association with risk groups or with moral degeneracy) from the range of lovers considered, in order to continue practicing unsafe sex with lovers chosen. Women in the study described collecting personal histories from their partners in order to identify and avert risks. However, these women did not always feel comfortable asking the questions relevant to their ideas of risk (e.g., about injection drug use or sex with men), and some did not discuss anything with their partners until after having had sex. The concepts of "trust" and "intuition" as methods of risk reduction were operative in these situations as well—if a general talk with a partner felt "right" and trust was established, then safer sex was considered unnecessary. In this case, as in the case of monogamous or committed relationships, emotional safety was equated with safety from transmission. However, other women reported feeling unable to disclose their past risk behaviors to potential partners *until* trust had been built to the point where discussing risk would not entail their being scrutinized and judged by their partners. Because of the additional stigmas in this community heaped on injection drug use and sex with men in the time of AIDS, women having engaged in these behaviors often feel unwilling to publicize them (Stevens and Hall, 1994b).

Temporary sexual abstinence and HIV testing represent other, less-frequently employed methods of attempted HIV risk reduction in the population of women who partner with women. Both are used to quell fears about HIV/AIDS, but do not necessarily lead to less risky behavior. In the Lyon-Martin study, testing largely figured as a justification for continuing unsafe or inconsistently safe sexual practices (If I'm still O.K. now, I must not be able to get HIV from what I've been doing) or for engaging in unsafe behaviors with another negative-tested person. Abstinence and HIV testing, when used as alternatives to committing to safer-sex practices, both illustrate a kind of moment-of-crisis style of thinking about HIV that appears incompatible with a sense of longer-term, more relaxed and livable approaches to HIV risk reduction. The panic that sometimes prompts testing or temporary abstinence can derive from a fatalistic attitude toward HIV, and seems to inhibit more personally directed and controlled problem-solving techniques. Panic seeks relief, which then allows for the putting off of realistic health concerns until the next bout of panic. While clinics offering HIV testing to women generally incorporate information in their pre- and post-test counseling about the temporal and other constraints of the test, even more emphasis must be placed on debunking the imagined function of the test for lesbians and bisexual women as a reassurance of past safety and a guarantee of future immunity.

MENTAL HEALTH CONCERNS FOR RISK REDUCTION

When examining the obstacles that women who have sex with women encounter in trying to negotiate and maintain the practice of safer sex, HIV educators will gain from an awareness of the connections between past experiences of physical, sexual, and emotional abuse and current risk behaviors. The SFDPH Prevention branch study found that 35 percent of the lesbian and bisexual sample had experienced physical abuse or battering, 13 percent in the past three years. Sixty-six percent reported having been emotionally abused, 37 percent in the past three years. Fifty-six percent of respondents had had suicidal thoughts, with 32 percent reporting them in the past three years. A full 40 percent of the sample had survived childhood sexual abuse or molestation (SFDPH Prevention, 1993). The relatively high presence of mental health stressors in the lesbian and bisexual female population likely influences sexual and drug-related behaviors in the direction of greater risk taking and less self-preservative action. Education and prevention targeting this group will need to strive to account for the functioning of these stressors, in addition to the functioning of stressors resulting from the combined cultural experience of misogyny, homophobia, racism, and class oppression. Ideally, education and prevention for lesbians and bisexual women will incorporate self-esteem building, acknowledgment of abuse-survival issues, general sexual communication skills-development, reinforcement of choice and agency in sexual encounters, and strategies for self-care in adversity.

SUPPORTING SAFER LOGICS WITH BETTER KNOWLEDGE

Of those women having sex with women who have changed some of their behaviors toward risk reduction, the inconsistent and contingent practice of safer sex still appears to be more common than a decidedly constant rule of safety. In negotiating their strategies for staying "semi-safe" (Stevens, 1993:11), women in this population continue to invoke the security of "monogamy," of "trust" relationships, of easily recognizable "risk groups," of special intuitive abilities, of spoken histories, and of other constructs that have proven unstable and contestable but that have been advanced as sites for real knowledge about HIV/AIDS in earlier phases of education and prevention. Women having sex with women have not been exempt from the influence of informational campaigns, but have been left to adapt the messages received to fit sexual practices and beliefs about personal and communal risk often incongruous with the instructional tone or content of prevention campaigns. These women's communities are, in fact, employing well-developed and fairly consistent *logics* of safety, which unfortunately can still lead to imperfect and inconsistent *practices* of safety.

The few existing studies of attitudes motivating the sexual and drug-related behaviors of women who have sex with women have convincingly demonstrated that the 100 percent rule is particularly hard for this population to accept as personally relevant. Rather than pouring all education and prevention resources for this population into attempts to increase its molding to an absolute model of safety, it would appear beneficial to improve the effectiveness of the models of prevention already established among women who have sex with women. What Stevens identifies as an ongoing, gradual process of behavioral change consisting of "episodes of choice" (Stevens and Hall, 1994b:22) must be enhanced by better, scientifically supported knowledge of the relative risks involved in the range of acts performed in women's sexual relations with each other. This population has been lacking in the kinds of specific information and tools needed to evaluate levels of risk attached to relevant behaviors, and has been targeted for education with the expectation that getting these women to follow instructions would not require any detailed grounding of those instructions in research.

"ALL OR NOTHING AT ALL": PROBLEMS WITH OVERLY DIRECTIVE EDUCATION

Walt Odets has questioned the benefits of the "100% safe 100% of the time" slogan for gay and bisexual men, whose real life behaviors also seem to differ from community-wide messages about the existence of new sexual norms and ethics—or a "Moral Majority," as established by the San Francisco AIDS Foundation (Odets, 1995). He argues that an unnecessarily strict, directive bent to HIV prevention education can lose the audience, for whom some safety measures would be acceptable but demands of absolute, airtight safety precautions prove discouraging and alienating from the whole objective of behavioral change. This analysis can also be appropriately applied to the population of women having sex with women. Women have historically, through the operations of societal, medical, and psychoanalytical programs dictating behaviors and expressions, been subjected to a great deal of investigation and correction in their casting as impure and disordering influences. Currently, women asked to evaluate their sexual behaviors with other women often express feelings of shame and inadequacy about their performance in relation to risk-reducing standards. Having fallen short of the standards of safety represented to them in the form of latex product promotions, and having little sense of the risk of certain activities relative to others, these women are likely to succumb to a sense of failure and confusion and to stop trying to reduce risk behaviors altogether.

In a move exemplary of its unique approach to HIV prevention, the Lyon-Martin peer education team made the recommendation that women intending to change only one sexual behavior with their female partners begin by wearing a latex glove. Cianna Stewart, one of the cofounders of the Peer Safer Sex Slut Team and currently a staff member at the Living Well Project Asian and Pacific Islander AIDS Services in San Francisco, explains the reasoning behind this emphasis on gloves in terms of the quick discouragement from safer-sex practices common among many women whose first attempts at safety involved dental dams. The Safer Sex Sluts weighed the advantages of an absolute model of safety against its disadvantages and decided to reinforce the more easily integrated and maintained risk-reductive behavior. Presumably, a person convinced that any method of safer sex can be a practicable, sensual, and normal aspect of everyday sexual behavior will be more receptive to learning about and adopting a range of safer behaviors.

The Lyon-Martin project encouraged women in one-on-one interviews and in group presentations to begin a gradual process of behavioral change, and to forgive themselves for past risk behaviors or occasional "slipping" from safety. The ideal of having a "clean slate" (Stevens and Hall, 1994b:22) from which one could decide always to practice safe behaviors was decentered in favor of a more practical view of achieving safety through constant episodical decisions about risk reduction. In these ways, the Safer Sex Sluts drew upon their closeness to the target audience without exploiting the punitive aspects of peer pressure. Relieving anxieties through humor, the community-based peer education undertaken by the Lyon-Martin team satirized the prescriptive tendencies of the "women's community" and debunked the labels around certain "types" of sex (e.g., "lesbian sex" or "heterosexual sex"). The team also made a point of challenging the authority of government statements about HIV and reminding their audiences of the potential motivating factors behind some of the received wisdom on HIV/AIDS. In order to assist women in thinking about and working on safety for positive and independent reasons, the project avoided scare and guilt tactics.

HIV prevention programs still need to make a conscious distinction between their aims and more familiar, sinister, and "sex-negative" attempts at regulating and homogenizing desires and their expressions. Otherwise, the abandoning of safer-sex objectives may be viewed as a revolutionary and liberatory act in a targeted population where membership already requires a willingness to live against the grain and in opposition to prescriptions for normative sexuality. Expressions by lesbians and bisexual women of revulsion toward the requirements of safer sex with women may reflect a feminist revulsion at the perception of further clinical controls being put on female sexual expressions: "It's sick—women are putting on gloves to touch other women. . . . No lesbian has gotten AIDS because she fist-fucked another woman. We're stigmatizing sexual practices" (Solomon, 1992:51). The drive for safer sexual norms has to come visibly from within the communities of women who have sex with women, and more specifically, who enjoy it.

Cianna Stewart argues that the main element of the team's success was its focus on the eroticization of safer-sex practices. She points out, as a source of strength for the project, its recruitment of peer educators from the sex industry. The call was put out through COYOTE and the social networks of female sex workers, and a team of women was selected for their sex-positivity, healthy exhibitionism, and enjoyment of talking frankly about sexual behaviors. They were chosen and intensively trained to be able to teach their audience how to practice safety not just "the right way," but in a more pleasurable way than they might have assumed possible.

IS SEX WORTH ITCHING FOR?
EVERYDAY APPROACHES TO SEXUAL HEALTH

In a fairly recent development in the attempts to translate the 100 percent message to populations of women sleeping with women, some health educators and activists have asserted that women need to practice safer-sex techniques with each other regardless of risk for HIV, because they can transmit a host of other STDs which could easily be prevented through the regular use of risk-reduction methods. Patton points out that lesbians need *sex* education anyway, and that safer-sex techniques provide general and vital information about how women have sex with women (Patton, 1991). When Jean Carlomusto follows Patton's explanation of the dental dam demonstration in the lesbian safer-sex video "Current Flow" (directed by Jean Carlomusto with Gregg Bordowitz for the Gay Men's Health Crisis Safer Sex Shorts, 1989) with the comment, "Yes, it's not just a question of HIV, but of a whole spectrum of illnesses that can result from the sexual exchange: yeast infections, chlamydia, and so on" (Patton, 1991:61–62), he reframes the dam question as one of generalized risk versus the maintenance of an all-over clean bill of sexual health. What he does not mention here is the evidence that vaginal infections both increase the chances of viral transmission and threaten the health of women whose immune systems may already be impaired by HIV (Chris, 1990). The potential for women to make informed choices about safer sex, through measuring their own risks and their threshold of tolerance for something as generally treatable as a yeast infection or chlamydia, gets overlooked entirely in this discussion of the urgency of basic sex education for women having sex with women. The prescription given here for the condition of lack of representation or reliable information presumes that latex should always precede specific information about HIV.

If the construct of safer sex, developed first in response to the HIV/AIDS epidemic, is to be expanded to include prevention of yeast infections (which can occur as a result of minor changes in diet, stress levels, hormone levels, and humidity as well as through sexual contact—they do not fit the usual definition of an STD), then the standard risk rhetoric of life-and-death sexual decisions must be challenged by a more focused and ordinary framework of sexual health priorities. This turn in the discussion around safer-sex techniques for women to use with other women seems to signal that the old "Is sex worth dying for?" approach to risk, which leaves no question as to its proper response, has been outmoded and exceeded by more complicated practices of sexual negotiation. While life-and-death choices have most often been determined within a logic of crisis necessitating the protection of the "greater good," choices about longer-term and everyday health concerns fall more readily into the realm of personal and communal values and resources. When advising women to use barriers with other women for general STD prevention, educators and health practitioners ought to be prepared to mention the range of STDs that can be transmitted through woman-to-woman sexual contact and to discuss the relative risk of certain activities for transmission of certain STDs, as well as the relative treatability of each STD. Women experienced in the care of yeast infections, chlamydia, and gardnerella, for example, might reasonably feel a great deal more concerned about the likelihood of their contracting and/or transmitting STDs like genital warts (linked to cervical cancer), herpes, or hepatitis B.

One of the most valuable ways to link HIV and STDs in prevention education targeting women who have sex with women may be to demonstrate, through discussing the variety of STDs commonly transmitted between women, the possibility of transmitting HIV through the same kinds of contact. The SFDPH study found that a full 5.4 percent of its participants tested positive for hepatitis B (SFDPH Surveillance, 1993), which is often used as an epidemiological marker for HIV. While the same group of women showed a significantly lower rate of HIV seropositivity, the presence of hepatitis B suggests that a higher prevalence of HIV among lesbian and bisexual women may be expected as they begin to have contact with more HIV positive partners. The Lyon-Martin peer educators brought up some of the more familiar STDs passed between women to make the point that lesbian and bisexual women are not somehow incapable of sexual transmission. In this way, the knowledge women already have about their risks and vulnerabilities in engaging in unprotected sex can be reinforced to bring HIV into focus as a personally relevant and comprehensible issue.

CONCLUSION: LESBIAN AND BISEXUAL WOMEN CONCEPTUALIZING SAFER SEX

In general, it seems that a workable approach to HIV education and prevention for the lesbian and bisexual women's population would need to account for the dominant perception of HIV/AIDS as having less-than-epidemic proportions in this population. Education mobilizing crisis logics and short-term emergency measures in women's communities may do much less good than education designed for long-term, gradual changes in sexual and drug-related behaviors. Odets discusses the dangers of telling a community to "Be Here for the Cure" (1995:3), when the chances of such a reprieve in our lifetimes from the HIV/AIDS epidemic grow constantly slimmer. Asking women to adopt "for now" prevention measures that they would not be able to maintain for their lifetimes makes failure to practice safety just a matter of time. It is critical to the health of this and other target populations that we study and publicize the relative risks of behaviors along with the most practical methods of risk reduction, and stop holding our breath for the moment when HIV no longer poses a threat.

Women who have sex with women especially need to be recognized in their risk for HIV through activities not culturally or epidemiologically accepted as "lesbian" behaviors. The minimal level of change made thus far in higher-risk behaviors among women who have sex with women suggests that HIV and AIDS may continue to rapidly grow as a public-health problem in this population. An emphasis on changing the behaviors that have been clearly established in other populations as routes of HIV transmission may be more practical and helpful at this point than an insistence on the use of barriers for woman-to-woman oral–genital contact. While the dental dam has not made the most convincing symbol of a movement for risk reduction, increased education for women about the use of other, less "lesbian-specific" safer-sex tools may succeed in effecting behavioral change. The aim expressed in the Lyon-Martin grant project title, "Women Dedicated to Demolishing Denial" (Stevens and Hall, 1994a: 1), could be continued through the formation of other projects that make it their point to reduce *all* forms of HIV risk impacting women who have sex with women.

The Lyon-Martin project established the importance of maintaining a consistent, long-term, integrated HIV-educational presence in the social and sexual environments of women who have sex with women, in order to situate safety on the level of a public, community issue. Women interviewed in the second year of this study testified to the influence of seeing the project around from week to week at clubs, bars, and community events. The appearance of this kind of outreach in the locations where women congregate was very new; and for some women who had not thought of HIV as a lesbian or bisexual women's issue, it was just the catalyst needed to make them reevaluate their assumptions of immunity. The private negotiations of women wanting to practice safer behaviors began to be reinforced by the larger discussions that developed out of group presentations and individual interviews with peer educators. The work of designing educational projects to reach this population has far to go, however, since the use of safer-sex techniques by women with other women still figures as the exception and not the rule, and it continues to be difficult even to bring up the issue of woman-to-woman safer sex. Lyon-Martin peer educators occasionally experienced animosity from women engaged in punishing the messenger of risk: "I resent that you are making such an issue about HIV in the lesbian community" (Stevens, 1993:19). This response suggests the role of willful ignorance in preserving the image of lesbian nonrisk.

At this point, communal denial has to be counteracted, in part, with a prevention approach to lesbians and bisexual women through their communities—utilizing existing networks, events, venues, and informational media to change the perception of risk for transmission in this population. Eventually, it may be more beneficial to challenge the very notions of community which have lent themselves so readily to the formation of socially bounded "risk groups" and blind spots. It is precisely those acts generally believed to put women at risk for HIV which are suppressed in the internally and externally produced image of the "lesbian community." In a social environment that many women experience as a pressure to identify as first lesbian, then a woman of color; first lesbian, then working class; first lesbian, then a woman who has sex with men and women; first lesbian, then a substance user or recovering addict; a concerted prevention effort is needed to uncover and address the higher-risk activities and cofactors characterizing women who have sex with other women.

Even when the methods and importance of safer-sex practices have been established clearly to individuals living in this population, there are obstacles to ensuring that safer sex occurs with their female partners. Many women interviewed in the Lyon-Martin project described being overwhelmed by the constant weighing of responsibility for safer sex on themselves alone (Stevens, 1993; Stevens and Hall, 1994a). Lesbian and bisexual advocates of the practice of safer sex find themselves fighting an uphill battle with women who are uninformed of their risk of HIV, are unconvinced of it, or are decidedly against the modification of their sexual practices to meet guidelines for safety. One woman contacted by the Lyon-Martin interviewers described having been shamed out of carrying her safer-sex supplies out to clubs when her female friends jeeringly noted her apparent eagerness for sex (Stevens, 1993). Other respondents also mentioned concerns about publicly overcommitting to and overpreparing for safer sex by purchasing their own supplies. Lesbians and bisexual women wanting to change their behaviors find themselves burdened with changing the behaviors and attitudes of their partners and even their friends in order to stick to their own resolutions.

Whether educators agree on the question of risk posed by woman-to-woman transmission, it would seem desirable to produce an environment of awareness among women who have sex with women of the presence and mobility of HIV in their communities and of the practice of several forms of safer sex, so that those women who have decided to make changes in their sexual behaviors are not met with fear, disgust, rage, ignorance, or other objections to their "making" HIV an issue. A blanket prescription for absolutely safe practices absolutely all of the time may never gain credibility in this population, but that does not necessarily constitute a loss for the side of education and prevention. Targeted educational efforts can productively use the habits women already have of making decisions about risk reduction in a context of negotiations continually strengthened by the influx of more specific and more reliable information about the transmission of HIV from women to their partners, with the result of empowering women knowledgeably to care for themselves and each other.

In view of the current scarcity of published research about woman-to-woman transmission and female fluid load factors, the experience of women involved in mixed HIV positive/negative or in positive/positive sexual relationships may prove to be an important source of information for women to use *now* for risk reduction in their exchanges with other women. The HIV positive member of a high-profile local magnetic lesbian couple (active in organizing women to respond to HIV and other health issues) recently made the surprising comment that no one had ever asked herself or her partner about how they have sex. Whether out of a sense of respect for privacy or a lack of ability to conceive that such couples could provide helpful models for safety, designers of education and prevention have not yet tapped the resources that magnetic couples have built in formulating their own practical strategies for preventing transmission. Instead of continuing to engage in the indefinite wait for personally relevant information that has characterized this population's relation to the epidemic thus far, women who have sex with women may take as a starting point the practices and frameworks for safety that female couples with one or two HIV positive member(s) have independently developed out of necessity and a very real and personal understanding of what it means to live with HIV.

APPENDIX: SAFER-SEX VIDEOS FOR WOMEN

"Safe Is Desire." San Francisco: Blush Entertainment Corp., 1993.
"She's Safe!" San Francisco: Frameline's Lesbian & Gay Cinema Collection,
    1994.
"Well Sexy Women." Produced by Pride Video Productions Ltd., England,
    1993. Distributed by Greenwood/Cooper Homevideo, Los Angeles.

NOTES

I am grateful to have had the assistance of Cianna Stewart, Roma Estevez, Claudia Goulston, Ami Becker, and Ann Smith in collecting information for this chapter. I am also indebted to Cynthia Gomez, Robert Schonberg, and Ann Smith for their close reading of its earlier drafts.

1. In the 1993 SFDPH "Health Behaviors" study, 37 percent of the sample of 483 lesbian and bisexual women reported knowing at least one woman living with HIV or AIDS, and an additional 14 percent reported knowing of at least one woman who has died of AIDS (SFDPH Prevention, 1993).

2. There is a newer exception in the Australian Glyde "Lollye" (from Kia-Ora Pacific Trading Party Limited); a wider, thinner latex shield designed by a woman for safer-sex purposes, but not widely available through retail sites or clinics in the United States. The Berkeley and San Francisco Good Vibrations stores carry the Glyde dam and also offer it on order through their store catalog, which greatly extends the possibilities for women in remote areas wishing to access safer-sex supplies. Good Vibrations currently has a site (with safer-sex and product information) on the *San Francisco Bay Guardian* electronic bulletin board, and will soon have its own World Wide Web site on the Internet.

3. Stanford University fellow Claudia Goulston has begun a study of HIV positive women to measure their fluid load factors in blood/plasma and in vaginal/cervical secretions. Her objective is to measure the viral load (of "free" virus in the fluid outside the cells, as well as the cell-associated load) in relation to the menstrual cycle and to chart any fluctuations that may take place as hormone levels shift. She will also examine the effects of hysterectomies and oral contraceptives on viral load, and will record the changes in load over time from HIV infection. Her data collection will include information about demographic makeup, sexual orientation, and risk factors of the participants. At the moment that this is written, she is

still in the process of recruiting her sample of fifty HIV positive women for this new study. She offered a description of her work plan in a phone conversation on June 2, 1995.

REFERENCES

Chris, Cynthia. (1990). Transmission Issues for Women. In *Women, AIDS, & Activism*, edited by Cynthia Chris and Monica Pearl, 17–25. Boston: South End Press.

Cohen, Judith B. (1993). HIV Risk among Women Who Have Sex with Women. *San Francisco Epidemiologic Bulletin* 9(4): 25–29.

Odets, W. (1995). The Fatal Mistakes of AIDS Education. *San Francisco Bay Times* 15(41): 3–7.

Patton, Cindy. (1991). Safe Sex and the Pornographic Vernacular. In *How Do I Look?*, edited by The Bad Object-Choices Collective, 31–63. Seattle: Bay Press.

Richardson, Diane. (1994). Inclusions and Exclusions: Lesbians, HIV, and AIDS. In *AIDS: Setting a Feminist Agenda*, edited by Lesley Doyal, Jennie Naidoo, and Tamsin Wilton, 159–170. Bristol, Pa.: Taylor & Francis.

San Francisco Department of Public Health, Prevention Services Branch, AIDS Office. (1993). Health Behaviors among Lesbians and Bisexual Women: A Community-Based Women's Health Survey. San Francisco: Department of Public Health.

San Francisco Department of Public Health, Surveillance Branch, AIDS Office. (1993). HIV Seroprevalence and Risk Behaviors among Lesbians and Bisexual Women: The 1993 San Francisco/Berkeley Women's Survey. San Francisco: Department of Public Health.

San Francisco Department of Public Health, Surveillance Branch, AIDS Office. (1995a). AIDS Surveillance Report. San Francisco: Department of Public Health.

San Francisco Department of Public Health, Surveillance Branch, AIDS Office. (1995b). HIV Seroprevalance Report. San Francisco: Department of Public Health.

Solomon, Nancy. (1992). Risky Business. *OUT/LOOK* 4(4): 46–52.

Stevens, Patricia E. (1993). HIV Risk Reduction for Three Subgroups of Lesbian and Bisexual Women in San Francisco—Year One: Project Evaluation Report. San Francisco: Lyon-Martin Women's Health Services.

Stevens, Patricia E., and Joanne M. Hall. (1994a). HIV Risk Reduction for Lesbians and Bisexual Women in San Francisco—Year Two: Mid-Year Evaluation Report. San Francisco: Lyon-Martin Women's Health Services.

Stevens, Patricia E., and Joanne M. Hall. (1994b). HIV Risk Reduction for Lesbians and Bisexual Women in San Francisco—Year Two: Year End Evaluation Report. San Francisco: Lyon-Martin Women's Health Services.

5

Red Clay and Rednecks: HIV Prevention in Rural Southern Communities

*Robert L. Barret and
Adam Robinson*

While the incidence of HIV infection in the state of North Carolina does not rival that of states like California, Texas, and New York, demographic information reveals that HIV is a mounting public-health issue. Data indicate that the problem is growing and will become more serious in the near future. Of the 4,803 AIDS cases reported as of March 1994, 1,780 (39%) appear in the white population and 2,618 (58%) occur in the African-American community. In spite of growing Hispanic and Asian communities, current seroprevalence data do not suggest that they are a priority audience as they are in other geographic areas.

Some years ago, in a presentation at the Lesbian and Gay Health Conference in San Francisco, we attempted to describe the kind of dynamics that accompany building support for an AIDS service organization in Jesse Helms's backyard. One of the truths about HIV work in North Carolina (and possibly other southern communities) is the need to adjust strategies to the conservative political reality in which we live. In our case, all HIV work demands careful strategizing.

This chapter will present some of the dynamics that surround effective HIV prevention work in North Carolina. Impressionistic rather than empirical, the chapter will review the environment in which HIV work is done, discuss the impact of HIV/AIDS consortia, present examples of some of the innovative approaches that are being used, and suggest what is needed for future work. Although not based specifically on empirical data, we believe the information we provide in this chapter is applicable to other southern states.

ENVIRONMENT

Data reinforce the appearance of a conspiracy of silence that allows communities to deny the existence of any threat from HIV disease. This is not all due to the presence of conservative political figures or even the so-called religious right. The primary factor that must be acknowledged is the unique ways oppression impacts rural and urban areas throughout the South.

For example, creating effective outreach programs to gay communities in small towns is complicated by the fact that gay people are largely invisible. Another complication is that not only do gay men fear oppression and violence if they do come out publicly, but they also accept an internal oppression that is often unconscious. Many gay men stop coming out because of the perception of an external threat, but also do not want to struggle with their own internalized homophobia. It is easier to not come out than to face one's own sense of shame and figure out how to overcome it. Such invisibility encourages the non-gay community to hold onto the stereotype of the gay man as effeminate and unstable and allows those who oppose gay rights to frame the debate in moral terms.

This conspiracy of silence infuses the gay community as well. At a recent monthly discussion group called Queer Conversations, when the topic of safe sex was selected, few had anything to say. Most sat in silence and when pushed to comment said simply, "I don't know anyone who has HIV disease, and I don't really want to talk about it." Anecdotal reports from counselors and psychotherapists indicate that many gay men continue to practice unsafe sex and also experience significant frustration because talking about their efforts to maintain safe-sex practices is not encouraged.

A similar attitude accompanies persons with HIV disease. In most southern communities, HIV continues to be seen as a moral issue. And being public about having HIV disease is still perceived as dangerous. One frequently mentioned barrier is that many fear the HIV-related shame that their families will face. The invisibility of the HIV-infected population is also enhanced by the fact that many go to nearby major population areas for medical care. Their statements go something like this: "I want to get the best care possible, and medical personnel in my town don't know anything about HIV treatment." This behavior leads local physicians and hospitals to respond to inquiries about HIV treatment with a statement like, "Oh, we have almost no HIV cases in our town. Few come in for treatment. It's really not a problem here."

Denial by the medical community plays right into the hands of politicians and other community leaders. Facing budgetary pressures that mimic those of big cities, the power structure is reassured that there is no HIV problem in their community and likes the idea that those who are infected will go to nearby cities for care. Given the kind of local boosterism that most of these communities embrace, admitting that there is an HIV problem in one's community is seen as an unnecessary liability, almost as something that is shameful to admit.

So, there is an absence of demand from the gay and HIV community that parallels a denial from the medical community, creating the illusion of "no problem" when it comes to HIV danger. There is an underlying problem that is frequently not acknowledged that also adds to the complexity of this issue. In the South, certain social traditions create rules that are often unstated but rigidly followed. One of those rules is that it is improper to acknowledge personal aspects of life in public. Talking about sex and illness, among other things, is a violation of that rule. This means that many who have grown up in these small towns do not have the language or the courage to talk about complicated topics like safe sex and HIV treatment. Frank discussions about sex in the public are rare, and most communities continue to believe that teaching teenagers about abstinence is all that is needed in a sound sex education program. In fact, there is a strong belief that risk-reduction strategies other than abstinence are immoral and should not be encouraged.

Further, HIV itself is seen as a moral issue in most of these communities. Creating prevention programs that seem to encourage behavior that is labeled immoral (sex alone, not to mention gay sex) demands solid approaches that help community leaders develop a new attitude towards HIV as a health issue.

Another complication is the tendency of national funding agencies to see the South in terms of its stereotype. Because southern communities are so backward and uninformed, it is not reasonable to spend hard won dollars to fund programs that may not have local support and may be very unsophisticated in terms of a final product. In many instances, southern communities have appeared near the top of proposed funding allocations but disappear on the final list. There are two reasons that often are given for the failure to fund: lack of sophistication and the negative political environment.

The presence of legislators like Jesse Helms is no small impediment. Because his office routinely requests copies of HIV-related materials, many funding agencies are reluctant to become involved in projects that might attract his attention. The last thing the CDC needs is to have Senator Helms waving explicit HIV prevention materials on the Senate floor. The fear of negative political consequences means a lack of resources for some southern states. Further, those who are charged to develop risk-reduction programs acquire a self-censoring attitude which limits their creativity and the final product; compared to materials developed in major metropolitan areas, risk-reduction pamphlets and other printed matter in the South lack the kind of explicitness that attracts attention.

Further, the power of the Christian church cannot be underestimated. Pastors and lay people in the church exercise much political influence, both directly and indirectly. An attitude exists, derived from traditional Protestant heritage, that has been institutionalized by present-day churches and can be seen in the actions of federal, state, and local politicians. The fact that some religious leaders use HIV/AIDS and the gay community to enhance their power is well known and understood by those in elective office. Even the current mayor of a large (450,000 population) city like Charlotte, North Carolina is not discouraged from making statements like, "We don't want to encourage a gay, lesbian, or bisexual presence in this community. We do not want to be another San Francisco. Gay people in Charlotte should go elsewhere." Politicians do not fear a backlash from making public statements like this one, and, in fact, often find renewed support for their candidacies as a result.

Garnering public support for the programs that do exist is also complicated. Politicians and funding agencies insist on the creation of citizen review panels to approve educational materials. Such panels get funding agencies and politicians off the hook and also seem to offer a method for prevention efforts to be supported. In practice, these panels constitute a huge impediment to the production of creative materials. First, not all of the targeted communities are represented. Gay men are routinely blocked from serving as members of these committees. Other minority presence is seen as essential, but placing a gay man in such a responsible position is simply too risky for state and local authorities. After all, in most southern states sodomy laws criminalize homosexuality, and appointing a known homosexual to a state review panel seems contrary to upholding the law. While the creation of a review panel could help ensure community support, the reality is that these bureaucratic hurdles discourage creativity and slow down the process of program implementation. Educators who are on the firing line trying to prevent HIV infection are disheartened by the kind of energy that is drained off seeking approval for every effort. An attitude of self-censorship emerges that dilutes the message. In one instance, a safe-sex pamphlet was not approved by a review panel until "Play Safe" was changed to "Play It Safe" and the word "fun" was deleted from the text. In another instance, a politician at the state level threatened to jeopardize the acceptance of federal funding after a supporter mailed him a gay-oriented prevention pamphlet. He also sent copies of the material to all state legislators in an effort to increase support for limited funding. Local HIV prevention educators were called away from their normal activities to respond to this crisis and began to operate in a climate charged with fear.

A unique challenge in the African-American community is the level of denial that exists within the black churches. Few ministers or congregations are willing to acknowledge that HIV is a threat and few educators are open to providing the kind of leadership that would enable programs to flourish. Segregation of whites and blacks results from natural social patterns. While all races are welcome at community events and bars, there is a tendency to socialize separately. Groups like Men of All Colors Together function with low participation from the white community, and, like the heterosexual world, there is little dating between races. Many African-American men who have sex with men do not identify as gay and will not utilize services that also have a gay clientele. This means that risk-reduction efforts in the African-American community must be designed to work in the specific settings.

The environment in which HIV prevention efforts occur is not one that encourages creative and explicit materials that are designed by individuals in the targeted communities. Local leaders feel secure in denying the presence of HIV, and local social institutions also fail to sound the alarm.

THE USE OF CONSORTIA

Under federal Ryan White legislation, HIV/AIDS consortia have been created throughout North Carolina. These collectives, usually housed in the urban centers, attempt to reduce the isolation reported by many who work in HIV service delivery and to break the silence about HIV that exists in rural areas. By providing personnel who travel out from the major cities and into rural counties to create local task forces, community-based education and service should improve.

What has been learned from this effort is that much patience is required. Because the political and social leadership is often in denial about the danger of HIV, there is much inertia that must be overcome. For example, in Union County, a task force was created in 1990 that included strong leadership. As this group met and acknowledged the problem, they floundered over what to do. When the local superintendent of the school system suggested having an art competition in the elementary schools, much enthusiasm was generated. All schools participated and the winning paintings were reproduced on billboards throughout the county. Opposition was stifled by the fact that the images had been created by innocent children, and an awareness of HIV as a local issue surfaced. But the leadership was not sure what to do next and never participated in long-range planning. Interacting with real people who have HIV disease was not seriously considered, and no one who was HIV infected came forward to put pressure on them to act in any specific way. Every meeting became an attempt to figure out what to do next, and there was little follow through to see that things got done. Finally, members quit attending and the task force disappeared. Today, a new task force has been formed that is being encouraged to formulate long-range plans and systems that insure follow-through.

Another activity of the consortia has been to educate physicians and nurses about HIV treatment and to survey clergy to see what kind of education efforts might succeed in garnering their support. Much of the HIV effort in these rural communities is designed to inform the leadership in the hope that support will follow for more direct action. By bringing together leadership from schools, churches, hospitals, and other community agencies like Hospice, a dialogue is created that might lead to more realistic and successful efforts.

An example of the impact of the consortia can be seen in the community of Gastonia. Gaston County is a typical rural county that had little awareness of HIV disease. The AIDS Council of Gaston County produced an effective brochure that includes photographs of local persons living with HIV disease. This effort personalized HIV throughout the county and has created more interest in prevention activities.

Yet often, local reaction indicates the kind of barriers that must be overcome. Recently the senior class in a rural high school in the Mooresville community planned an AIDS awareness week. One part of their program included having a person with AIDS speak to the student body. Parents started calling the principal to complain and eventually the program was canceled. School administrators were not certain of support from school board members, and, in spite of major media coverage, fear and lack of information was reinforced.

This conservative stifling of efforts also occurs through calculated effort. The Charlotte community identified the need to reduce teen pregnancy and STD rates. Collaborations of agencies have begun a process to change the school curricula to address the needs of the most high-risk teenagers. Conservative opposition has taken the form of orchestrated inclusion on advisory panels. One such community panel includes members that advocate for abstinence-only programs. One of these members attached a list of "further recommendations" to their report which included the recommendations that the curricula not address issues of sexual orientation at all. Her additions were discovered to be her own rather than the committee's; however, the incident illustrates the planful way conservative community members try to pursue their agendas in spite of sound health education guidelines.

PROGRAMS THAT WORK

There are risk-reduction efforts that succeed in spite of the atmosphere that characterizes rural southern communities. Familiar efforts like bar brigades, pamphlets in areas where at-risk populations gather, and condom distribution are common. And, in one more liberal community, the local school board approved condom distribution at the area high school. There are other instances where creative and effective programs have been developed.

In Charlotte, there is an annual Youth and AIDS conference that evades the pressure to censor. By inviting seventh and eighth graders to attend voluntarily and scheduling on the weekend, planners do not have to have school administrative approval. Local AIDS service organizations, the Red Cross, and some civic service organizations cosponsor the two-day event, where over 150 youths learn about HIV disease and prevention measures in an atmosphere that embraces rather than stifles sexuality. By not being an *official* school event, the conference remains free of the political scrutiny and pressure that school boards can bring to bear. However, in a particularly southern way, school officials "look the other way" and do not exercise their gate-keeping tendency. Local media publicize and support the event, and few question its appropriateness. The result is a growing number of students who have been informed and have learned ways to function as peer helpers.

Outreach on college campuses takes the familiar form of AIDS awareness weeks that are composed of various programs both in and out of residence halls. Because attendance at these events is low, residence-life staff and student development offices have taken to including HIV prevention education as a part of the required freshman orientation program. Efforts on the many church-affiliated college campuses are more difficult.

Most successful have been panels of persons living with HIV disease, either as special programs or as in-class presentations. In general, these attempts rely on the interest and commitment of one or more individuals who are willing to risk getting in trouble with administrators because they know students are sexually active and candidates for HIV infection. At a recent presentation on a church-related campus of 600 students, over 100 students and three administrators attended. Following this presentation, condoms were placed on the open shelves in the college bookstore. One administrator commented, "I know we will get some flack from members of our Board of Directors about this. I can live with that. Frankly, I am more concerned that few students will have the courage to buy condoms where they might be seen by others. When it comes to sexual activity, the attitude seems to be one of don't ask, don't tell."

Educators in Greensboro developed an initiative to reduce HIV transmission in the African-American community. Youth Protectors of Life (YPOL) recruits African-American youths in churches to become involved in HIV efforts throughout the community. The first step involved having youths participate in nonthreatening projects that churches could sponsor in the spirit of compassion. Gathering food that was distributed by local food pantries created an initial involvement that provided food that was distributed to persons living with HIV disease. Using the church as a base, YPOL opened doors that, eventually, older church members walked through. Now whole congregations have learned about YPOL and the local AIDS Service Organization (ASO).

In the western part of North Carolina, the gay African-American community is very isolated from mainstream gay activities and misses out on information provided in gay bars and in the gay media. Their social life centers around private parties, often involving drag themes and drug use. Needle sharing and sex between men are frequent behaviors that are rarely acknowledged. In response, the local ASO has recruited non-white peer educators, who attend the parties and encourage the hosts to become advocates for risk reduction. The result has been safer-sex themed drag shows that do not use the words gay or bisexual but educate about the risk of HIV infection and effective prevention.

Rural men experience isolation by their distance from organized gay community activities. Personal ads, placed in the two major gay community newspapers that are distributed statewide, provide a way to meet other gay men. One ASO reads the ads and sends the men who list addresses packets of HIV prevention materials, condoms, and water-based lubricant samples. These safer-sex "gift packets" have been very popular with recipients, primarily because of the erotic and explicit brochures. The packets have been mailed to communities throughout the state, providing solid information to men who might not otherwise be reachable. Some have contacted the ASO for more information.

Other men, who may be isolated by their sexual desires and behaviors, frequent erotic bookstores where they find men seeking sexual contacts. One stereotype of these men is that of men in heterosexual marriages who also desire sex with men. The reasons for seeking anonymous sexual encounters are complex, but include a belief that they do not deserve or will never be capable of more intimate sexual relationships with men. This cruising behavior is characterized by personal conflict and often leads to sexual behavior that is unsafe. Erotic bookstore outreach is one way HIV prevention provides information to this population. Included along with safer-sex information are gay affirmative pamphlets that seek to erode some of the shame of sex between men and hopefully begin or support the process of coming out. In North Carolina, the ASOs that do this work have a simple strategy. The staff of the bookstore is trained in HIV basics with a focus on HIV prevention. They are supplied with erotic posters and brochures that can be displayed in the store. Eventually, they are asked to distribute safer-sex packets to their customers. The specific method of distribution depends on the wishes of the store management. One store gives a safer-sex packet to every man who purchases male-oriented erotica. Some staff have become active in encouraging their patrons to be safe and others have expressed their homophobia by refusing to participate. It is hoped that this approach will change the setting to one that nurtures healthy attitudes rather than reinforcing a kind of shame that locks many in positions that guarantee dissatisfaction and leads to unsafe sex.

The shame exists for heterosexual men as well. They rarely call the local AIDS hotline, but have found a more anonymous and psychologically safer venue for discussion. Computerized bulletin board systems (BBSs) provide an opportunity to chat with other people through typed text. A regional erotic BBS has developed and recognized the need for HIV education to be part of the service provided. Men, described by their volunteer HIV educator as "unsophisticated Bubbas," type their chatty questions to her. The format allows for explicit and informal education to take place where it rarely did before.

Other efforts are directed at African-American women. In local public housing projects, women are invited to tupperware party–style house parties to learn about AIDS prevention. They discuss experiences they have with initiating or maintaining risk-reduction strategies. The creation of local social support is hoped to encourage the application of knowledge to actual risk reduction.

This same type of work occurs in correctional facilities for women. The program is entirely run by the local ASO, with cursory approval of the correctional system. Attitudes of guards and administration seem the chief barrier. The ASO had hoped to give condoms to the women to have when they leave the prisons. Officials refuse to allow the distribution, arguing that condoms are contraband even in all-women facilities. The program is successful, though, in bringing people with HIV who have themselves been incarcerated to the current inmates.

While these programs may seem tame by standards typically found in HIV epicenters, they function because they acknowledge community barriers and reach hard to find populations.

CONCLUSION

The struggles of prevention work in North Carolina illustrate many of the uniquely southern dynamics that inhibit HIV education. In response to these barriers, strategies have emerged that succeed. The general denial of need is being countered by Consortia that strive to cultivate local leadership in rural areas. Support for prevention work is gradually developing outside the cities of North Carolina.

Sometimes the political interference can be avoided by providing alternative venues for education. These approaches (e.g., the Youth and AIDS Conference) can be outside political jurisdictions and yet serve the same systems that would not endorse them. Churches are similarly restrained by attitudes that inhibit education. Nonetheless, their history of care and compassion can be capitalized upon to develop trust between the church and local ASOs. This "foot-in-the-door" technique can become an invitation to work with the churches rather than against them.

Relationships are harder to create across distances. Sometimes education can occur long distance by utilizing preexisting methods of communication (such as personal ads and computerized bulletin board systems). Psychological distance is harder to overcome. For many people at high risk for HIV, their own risk behaviors are far from integrated into their rational spheres. When educators are able to join with them, creating an environment that is nurturing of self-esteem and integration, a step toward health has been taken. As educators, we must overcome our own oppressions (our classism, racism, and homophobia) to be able to help our target audiences dispel some of the oppression that leads to silence and erodes regard for health. Only in this way will HIV prevention in North Carolina reach the level and impact that will be necessary to quell this virus.

6

HIV/AIDS Education and Prevention in the Asian American and Pacific Islander Communities

Michael Jang

The focus of HIV/AIDS prevention and education in the United States has shifted from the general public to high-risk populations. This shift is based on the assumption that large federal and state HIV/AIDS campaigns have increased the general public's awareness of HIV/AIDS, and, indeed, National Center for Health Statistics surveys have confirmed the effectiveness of these campaigns.

In the case of Asians and Pacific Islanders, immigration will continue to be the major cause of growth of this population. It is estimated that there will be an additional four to six million Asians and Pacific Islanders immigrating to the United States by the year 2000. It is evident that there will be a continued need to increase the knowledge and awareness about HIV/AIDS for the newly arrived immigrants during the remainder of the 1990s.

The Association of Asian/Pacific Community Health Organizations (AAPCHO) is a national network of community health centers that serve the Asian/Pacific Islander populations. The association includes Asian Health Services in Oakland, California; Asian Pacific Health Care Venture in Los Angeles; Chinatown Health Clinic in New York City; International District Community Health Center in Seattle; Kokua Kalihi Valley and Waianae Coast Comprehensive Center in Honolulu; North East Medical Services in San Francisco; and South Cove Community Health Center in Boston.

These centers provide bilingual and bicultural services to primarily low-income clients. The centers' service delivery operates on a community health-center model that emphasizes primary health care and health promotion and disease prevention. In 1989, AAPCHO received a grant from the Centers for Disease Control and Prevention to improve the delivery of HIV/AIDS education to Asian/Pacific Islander immigrants in the United States. The purpose of the Asian/Pacific Islander HIV/AIDS Resource and Training Project is to prevent the spread of HIV/AIDS among service populations of Asian/Pacific Islander health centers and to increase awareness of HIV/AIDS as an important health concern in those communities.

Central to the HIV/AIDS education model developed by AAPCHO is the need for culturally appropriate and culturally derived educational approaches that take into account the great heterogeneity of the Asian/Pacific Islander community and that challenge the myth of Asians as "the good minority."

Asian Americans and Pacific Islanders constitute a wide range of separate and culturally distinct groups, but they are usually combined for reporting purposes. Even these broad nomenclatures underscore the differences between the two. *Asian American* is a term applied to persons in the United States "having origins in any of the original people of the Far East." *Pacific Islander* is a more ambiguous term that includes persons who have origins in a group of predominantly small island nations that have a close relationship with the United States (i.e., Guam, American Samoa, the Republic of Palau, the Republic of the Marshall Islands, the Commonwealth of the Northern Mariana Islands, and the Federated States of Micronesia), Native Hawaiians, and others who are immigrants or long-standing American citizens whose ancestors came from South Pacific islands.

Asian Americans/Pacific Islanders compose the third-largest minority group in the United States after African Americans and Hispanics or Latinos. They are also the fastest growing community of color. The diversity of the Asian American/Pacific Islander population is extraordinary. Federal data collectors currently recognize the following subcategories: Chinese, Japanese, Hawaiian, Filipino, and Other Asian/Pacific Islanders. The last category alone includes over thirty-nine different nationalities. Collectively, they speak over

100 languages and dialects. Moreover, there can be great cultural, social, economic, and political differences within specific ethnic groups, as well as between dissimilar ethnic groups; for example, between fifth-generation Chinese Americans and new immigrants.

After decades of intermarriage, the Pacific Island populations are a mixture of racial backgrounds. Individuals often identify with the ethnic culture that is dominant in their household, and when this fact is not taken into consideration, demographic data that report race and ethnicity as only one choice will not reflect accurate information for a population as racially and ethnically diverse as the Pacific Islanders. For example, the 1990 U.S. Census reported approximately 138,000 self-identified Hawaiians residing in Hawaii, while the Hawaii Department of Health's annual Health Surveillance Program estimated that, by 1986, there were already nearly 205,000 residents of Hawaiian ancestry.

EPIDEMIOLOGY

Of the 401,749 total AIDS cases in the United States through June 1994, the Centers for Disease Control and Prevention reported that 2,706 (0.7%) were Asian Americans/Pacific Islanders. The Asian American/Pacific Islander male-to-female ratio of AIDS cases is approximately eleven to one. In 1991, Asian Americans/Pacific Islanders had an annual AIDS case rate of 3.7 per 100,000 population.

When exposure categories are examined, it is apparent that the HIV epidemic among Asian Americans/Pacific Islanders is still in the early stages. Of the AIDS cases in the Asian American/Pacific Islander community, 74 percent were men who have sex with men, compared with 58 percent for all races. Among the pediatric cases, 16 percent have been in children with hemophilia, and 37 percent were due to transmission of HIV through blood transfusions or blood products. All these categories are strikingly higher than the national averages and resemble data collected at the beginning of the epidemic in other racial groups.

Conversely, only 4 percent of all AIDS cases in adult and adolescent Asian Americans/Pacific Islanders have been due to injection drug use. Furthermore, only 47 percent of pediatric cases have been due to perinatal transmission from a mother at risk for HIV. These rates are much lower than the national averages. Again, this is reminiscent of epidemiologic data obtained in the early years of the HIV/AIDS epidemic for other groups.

Several researchers found, in studies of knowledge, attitudes, and behaviors (KAB) of Asians and Pacific Islander populations, that HIV/AIDS knowledge scores among immigrant groups are low and that myths about HIV/AIDS transmission are still prevalent. In a study of HIV/AIDS KAB in San Francisco's Filipino community in 1990, common misconceptions about modes of HIV/AIDS transmission included the belief that HIV/AIDS is caused by sharing toothbrushes (66%), by needles used for vaccinations or laboratory tests (57%), by receiving a blood transfusion after 1985 (54%), by donating blood (42%), and through mosquito bites (35%).

NATIONAL PREVENTION PROGRAMS

Programs for the prevention and care of HIV/AIDS among Asian Americans/Pacific Islanders have only recently been developed and funded. Currently, a number of organizations are working to meet the HIV/AIDS service needs of the Asian American/Pacific Islander communities. On the national level, organizations such as the Asian American Health Forum, the Association of Asian/Pacific Community Health Organizations, and the National Asian/Pacific American Families Against Substance Abuse are working to raise awareness about the HIV/AIDS service needs of the Asian American/Pacific Islander communities. This chapter focuses on the experience of one of these national programs—the Association of Asian/Pacific Community Health Organizations (AAPCHO).

The first phase of the CDC-funded program focused primarily on the initial training of AAPCHO staff, developing HIV/AIDS education materials, and enhancing information dissemination networks. This initial phase allowed program staff to learn the skills and to develop the educational materials needed to pursue the objectives for the following years.

During year two, training of the AAPCHO staff reinforced the skills learned in phase one. The program staff coordinated the training of AIDS liaisons at AAPCHO centers and the increased utilization of AAPCHO's standardized education and testing curriculum. Program staff began community outreach, distributing HIV/AIDS prevention information to staff, clients, and communities through health fairs, Asian media, and one-to-one counseling.

During year three, program staff provided basic training to clinic staff, as well as advanced training to staff with previous basic skills training. Outreach efforts continued, targeting churches, schools, patients, and senior citizens. Program staff translated an HIV/AIDS health education video to Laotian, Cambodian, and Japanese. The staff reviewed existing HIV/AIDS materials and developed a comprehensive packet of multilingual materials for youth. The staff also developed an evaluation methodology to be used in the final year.

During year four, the program staff continued reinforcement training of clinic staff on advanced HIV/AIDS skills and culturally appropriate program evaluation. In addition, program staff trained AAPCHO staff and Junior Health Educators on basic HIV/AIDS information. The program staff conducted HIV/AIDS prevention outreach to community members through radio broadcast programs and the "Behind the Mask" video rental. Staff developed additional HIV/AIDS information materials, such as a fact sheet on AIDS, STDs, and Hepatitis B in English, Vietnamese, Chinese, Tagalog, and Samoan, and translated the "Behind the Mask" video to a Mien version.

The final year consisted of summarizing the education materials and program models. The staff continued to train community members and center staff. Community outreach through radio and TV programs took place. And, finally, program staff evaluated the free video-rental project. What follows is a summary of that analysis.

NATIONAL AND REGIONAL TRAINING

In March 1992, AAPCHO developed and implemented training workshops in which representatives of Asian and Pacific Islander centers (Asian Health Services, Asian Pacific Health Care Venture, Chinatown Health Clinic, International District Community Health Center, Kokua Kalihi Valley Community Center, North East Medical Services, and South Cove Community Health Center) and their community counterparts participated to increase their skills and knowledge of HIV/AIDS prevention. In addition, the centers conducted in-service training sessions for their staff. The training topics included adult learning theory, training methods and outreach strategies, updates on trends and research findings on HIV/AIDS, sexuality and HIV/AIDS, physiological and psychosocial issues surrounding HIV/AIDS, program development and evaluation, and other skills necessary for clinic staff and health educators to provide effective community education.

In March 1993, AAPCHO developed and implemented training workshops in which representatives of the same Asian and Pacific Islander health centers (including the Waianae Coast Comprehensive Health Center) and their community counterparts participated. The workshop participants identified and documented successful and unique HIV/AIDS prevention and education models for Asian and Pacific Islanders; increased knowledge in culturally sensitive approaches for HIV/AIDS prevention and education; improved skills in staff training, community outreach and education, education information dissemination, and media approach for HIV/AIDS prevention;

and increased knowledge in HIV/AIDS prevention specifically related to women, youths, and legal, immigration, and ethical issues.

Community HIV/AIDS Presentations and Workshops

The participating centers provided HIV/AIDS education in seven cities within five states for Asian/Pacific Islander communities. Participating centers conducted these presentations and workshops in community health clinics, local schools, community colleges, and community agencies. Participants in these workshops learned information about HIV/AIDS, including how the virus is transmitted, and how individuals can prevent the spread of HIV. In addition, the curriculum emphasized Asian and Pacific Islander specific risk factors and their vulnerability to HIV/AIDS. Such risk factors include both single and married males frequenting massage parlors, and prostitutes and clients from the "Golden Triangle," who inject heroin, sharing needles.

Production and Distribution of "Behind the Mask"

AAPCHO developed and produced culturally sensitive education videos for Asians and Pacific Islanders. The video "Behind the Mask" focuses on values and themes that are particularly important to these communities—for example, everybody can get HIV, not just gays; and if one becomes HIV positive, the family can play a supportive role. The video consists of an all Asian/Pacific Islander cast and is available in nine Asian/Pacific languages, as well as English. The nine languages include Cantonese, Cambodian (Khmer), Korean, Laotian, Mandarin, Mien, Samoan, Tagalog, and Vietnamese. AAPCHO distributed a total of 981 copies of the video to health centers, community agencies, public-health organizations, and other agencies. AAPCHO and the Center for Southeast Asian Refugee Resettlement in San Francisco jointly initiated a free video-rental project at seven video stores in that city's Tenderloin District.

Development, Collection, and Dissemination of AIDS Information

The participating centers developed culturally appropriate HIV/AIDS prevention materials for community education. AAPCHO searched for existing materials in Asian/Pacific languages and English. AAPCHO distributed these materials to the centers for review and revision. Accurate translations were printed and distributed to the centers. Community and center clientele received the HIV/AIDS materials, as well as Hepatitis B and STD information, through community health fairs, education outreaches, and education workshops.

Radio Broadcasts, Television Programs, and Newspaper Articles

AAPCHO and the participating centers used radio, television, and newspapers to reach a greater population base. The project staff produced and distributed a half-hour radio program focusing on Asians and Pacific Islanders and AIDS to radio stations for airing throughout the nation. Television programs discussing HIV/AIDS were broadcasted. AAPCHO and the centers also published public-health and newspaper articles.

ACCOMPLISHMENTS

AAPCHO programs have been quite successful. The following is a summary of the significant accomplishments.

National and Regional Training

- Five culturally appropriate training curricula were developed.
- 360 center staff and their community counterparts were trained on HIV/AIDS at the beginning, intermediate, and advanced levels.
- HIV/AIDS knowledge increased between 14 and 39 percent from the training.
- Seven AAPCHO center project liaisons completed project planning and evaluation workshops.

Community HIV/AIDS Presentations and Workshops

- 6,210 community members participated in education workshops at seven participating centers.
- Pre-/post-tests indicated that knowledge increase ranged from 10 to 35 percent, and greater than 80 percent knowledge competency on the information presented to the participants.

Production and Distribution of "Behind the Mask"

- The video "Behind the Mask" was produced in English and translated into nine Asian and Pacific Islander languages. This video received a 1991 honorable mention at the American Film and Video Festival.

- More than 450 videos have been rented free by community members through an innovative method of outreaching to community video stores.
- 494 complementary copies of the video were provided to the centers and other community agencies, and 487 copies were sold at a nominal cost.

Development, Collection, and Dissemination of AIDS information

- AAPCHO and the centers developed and reviewed over fifty pieces of HIV/AIDS educational materials. These materials were translated into over ten Asian and Pacific Islander languages.
- Over 72,114 HIV/AIDS education and prevention information materials and brochures have been distributed to community members.

Radio Broadcasts, Television Programs, and Newspaper Articles

- Over 900 cassettes of the radio documentary produced by AAPCHO, "Behind the Mask: AIDS in the Asian Pacific Community," were distributed to radio stations. The program received a 1990 National Federation of Communication and Broadcast honorable mention for news and public-affairs programming.
- An estimated 178,250 community members have been reached through radio, television programs, and articles furnished by the centers.

Collaboration and Technical Assistance

- AAPCHO and the centers established collaboration with and provided technical assistance to over 200 other agencies, including local health departments and community-based health organizations.

Project Evaluation

- A culturally appropriate and sensitive evaluation methodology has been developed to measure the effectiveness and document the impact of this project.

WHAT HAVE WE LEARNED?

Staff and administrators of AAPCHO have learned many important tips to keep in mind when providing HIV/AIDS education and prevention to the Asian/Pacific Islander communities. Among the most salient are the following.

Staffing and Training

Most center personnel believe that staffing is inadequate for the amount of education activities conducted. Several centers received additional resources or supportive services from their state or local health agencies for HIV/AIDS prevention activities. These additional funds provided for staff to specialize in HIV/AIDS education. In most other clinics, health educators simply added HIV/AIDS education to their many other responsibilities. Most health educators in the AAPCHO centers were bicultural as well as bilingual. Many of the educators had also worked as health educators in their country of origin. Careful staff recruitment contributed to the centers' ability to reach and educate the target populations.

Current research continuously provides new information on HIV/AIDS education. For example, new opportunistic infections are being added to the list of AIDS-related diseases. New experimental drugs are being added for AIDS treatment. And new data from the prevention literature help to develop promising education strategies. It is recommended that AAPCHO prepare a series of HIV/AIDS education updates that denote, by target group, the basic, up-to-date information that should be covered in any HIV/AIDS education effort. In addition, the AAPCHO centers should ensure that all HIV/AIDS staff training throughout the centers meet minimum standards regarding current and accurate HIV/AIDS information.

A wider dissemination and sharing of educational interventions among centers is needed on an ongoing basis. This does not necessarily mean dissemination of "model programs," but rather an ongoing exchange among contractors, where they can share what does and does not work. Any dissemination of successful programs should be done with caution. Centers should be encouraged to explore and examine their own communities before adopting, in total, any program from a different community.

Community Education

In many Asian and Pacific Islander cultures, sexual matters are not openly discussed among strangers, especially between males and females. This cultural value can cause uneasiness and inhibit open discussions among participants. Several centers therefore provide separate classes for males and females to ease the participants' discomfort and encourage more interaction between the two.

In contrast to the general population where HIV/AIDS information is often provided in work settings and large community meetings at churches or clubs, the immigrant and refugee populations are best reached through formal educational settings, such as English as a Second Language classes, community colleges, or health clinics where ancillary health services and education take place. One health clinic serving primarily Native Hawaiians conducts outreach by identifying natural groups and providing education in natural settings. For example, this clinic often conducts HIV/AIDS education in homes or at beach parties, where friends gather informally.

Media Communication

Because of the high growth of Asian and Pacific Islander populations in the United States and the concentration of these populations in large urban states, radio and television markets have opened up in large metropolitan areas. For example, in California, programs in Chinese, Tagalog, Vietnamese, Japanese, anc ,ambodian are available through UHF and cable stations. Many of the cable programs produced and presented through International Television are available to major television markets in Hawaii, as well as mainland United States. The opening of radio and television markets provides an opportunity to conduct public media campaigns for the Asian and Pacific Islander communities. Staff from the San Francisco center appeared on Chinese programs to talk about HIV/AIDS. Other health centers also use radio or television as an HIV/AIDS education outreach strategy. To date, there is little research to confirm the types of Asian and Pacific Islander messages that are effective. However, on the basis of health campaigns in Asia and a few antismoking campaigns in California, messages based on a strong family and caring of family members, with appropriate cultural images, appear to be effective.

The initial dissemination of the video "Behind the Mask" through local video stores was slow. The video store owners were reluctant to shelve and promote the free rental of the video, fearing that it would jeopardize their business. One project found the target community received the message more effectively when local community health-outreach workers distributed the video. Others found that better publicity, and specifically informing community members of the availability of the HIV/AIDS prevention video, was important in promoting community awareness of the HIV/AIDS threat.

When launching a Saturday Samoan-language radio program called "You and Your Choices: Making Your Health a Priority," health educators at Kokua Kalihi Valley found that Samoan custom calls for apologies when using HIV/AIDS messages that discussed certain body parts or sex. They also noted the importance of the family and church when communicating health messages. In addition, the health educators developed terminology to express "risk" and other words or ideas that are not part of the Samoan language.

Most centers agreed that there is a shortage of professionally designed educational materials targeted to the Asian and Pacific Islander communities. Inadequate funding is the major cause for this shortage. The centers believe the important issues in the development of effective messages through pamphlets and posters are the quality of the art work and layout, the clarity of the message about HIV/AIDS, the severity of the HIV/AIDS problem being portrayed, the simplicity of the wording, and the appropriateness of the language. The problems with educational material development will become more acute as more Asian and Pacific Islander agencies receive funding from other sources. The process of producing Asian and Pacific Islander educational materials can be implemented systematically, through grants and contracts to agencies with expertise in the design and production of multicultural health education materials. It is more efficient to have experts produce attractive materials after addressing the design needs and criteria with educational agencies who are serving Asian and Pacific Islander populations.

Community-Oriented Primary-Care Model

Community-oriented primary care combines the traditional principles of primary care and public health in the planning and delivery of health-care services. The participating health centers provide primary-care services to a defined community, coupled with systematic efforts to identify and address the major health problems of that community through effective modification in both the primary-care services and other appropriate community health programs. The model has three components. First, the practice or service program should be actively engaged in primary care that is comprehensive in nature, accessible to those targeted, and accountable for service delivery. The second component of the model necessitates that the practice or service program define a community and take responsibility for that community's health and health care. The third component involves the process by which the major health problems of the community are addressed.

AAPCHO found that community-oriented primary-care programs are more effective if indigenous, bicultural service providers are used in the health practice. These professionals understand and identify with the recipients' problems and concerns to a greater degree than professionals who do not speak the appropriate language or understand the cultural values, traditions, attitudes, beliefs, or practices of the targeted community.

Collaboration and Technical Assistance

Major strengths of the Asian/Pacific National HIV/AIDS Resource and Training Project included collaboration and technical assistance with both private and public agencies throughout the United States. AAPCHO and its centers worked with national HIV/AIDS organizations; public-health agencies at the federal, state, and local levels; educational institutions; as well as foreign national health organizations. At the seven local centers, the project provided technical assistance and collaborated with ninety-four community-based organizations (CBOs). The majority of the CBOs and public-health agencies worked through collaboration, while the educational institutions and other agencies primarily received technical assistance.

Examples of collaboration included the development of the video "Behind the Mask," where CBOs and media organizations were asked to participate in focus groups, to critique the scripts, and to work together on the filming of the video. AAPCHO center staff provided technical assistance to their targeted Asian and Pacific Islander communities, as well as other local and state agencies working in the HIV/AIDS area. The amount and quality of technical assistance and collaboration given by this project exemplify the ability of the health centers to serve and advocate for its target population.

CONCLUSION AND RECOMMENDATIONS

The purpose of the Asian Pacific National HIV/AIDS Resources and Training Project is to provide HIV/AIDS education to the communities that are served by the AAPCHO centers. The evaluation staff were faced with the task of attempting to evaluate these programs and extracting from them elements which either assisted or hindered program success.

The evaluation team found that AAPCHO and its health centers met and often exceeded the objectives as specified in the Centers for Disease Control and Prevention contract. In addition, the AAPCHO centers accomplished their many objectives in a cost-efficient manner. That is, the centers were able to reach and educate their monolingual clients within the clinic setting as well as perform outreach to other monolingual community members. AAPCHO centers appear to be an excellent vehicle to deliver HIV/AIDS education, especially to hard-to-reach immigrant populations.

Despite the fact that the AIDS epidemic is more than ten years old and that funding for HIV/AIDS education for Asian and Pacific Islanders has been provided in this country since 1986, the evaluation team found that a number of "old" health education lessons are still highly relevant. Some of these include the following:

1. No single educational strategy is able to do the entire job; several are needed.
2. Effective educational interventions include an intimate knowledge of the target populations.
3. Educational intervention development requires careful planning, analysis, literature review, and a theoretical basis.
4. Programs without adequate provision for evaluation offer only limited guidance for future education and prevention programs.

Many people continue to believe that Asians and Pacific Islanders, as well as other minorities, refuse to acknowledge that AIDS is a multicultural problem. In fact, we have now learned that the Asian and Pacific communities could not and did not relate to the same type of AIDS media campaign being used to inform the general public. Thus, Asians, Pacific Islanders, and other minority communities are often (ironically) blamed for their lack of education. It has been mistakenly assumed that everyone understands health issues in the same context, despite the fact that the health education literature repeatedly indicates that issues of well-being are best approached in a cultural context.

Salient educational issues for Asians and Pacific Islanders include the following:

1. Keep it basic, at least at first; whether in English or one's native language, messages that are too elaborate are bound to tax someone's linguistic abilities (presenter or participant), comprehension, time, or attention span.
2. Repeat messages; educators may have to repeat messages several times or build in some leeway for incremental learning.
3. Include as many relevant learning approaches as possible for the audience—graphic, spoken word, video, written word, physical interaction, and so forth.

The National AIDS Minority Information and Education program accomplished its stated objectives, including staff training, community outreach, information dissemination, and mass-media information outreach. The key to AAPCHO's programmatic success was the intergration of indigenous and bicultural service providers into the community-oriented primary-care model. AAPCHO enhanced service providers' ability to understand and identify with the clients' cultural values, traditions, beliefs, and practices, and amplified the rate which the HIV/AIDS messages were comprehended. This program contributed a necessary component for building the knowledge and awareness of HIV/AIDS in the present and newly arriving Asian and Pacific Islander populations.

7

Evolution of a Model of Popular Health Education for Environmental Change in the Latino Community

Susana Hennessey Touré and
Cassandra Hernández Vives

Doña Cata, an eighty-six-year-old Latina, approaches the altar of her local church and addresses the congregation about an upcoming rally. A group of Latinos work together to develop and implement a local food cooperative. A thirty-four-year-old monoligual Spanish-speaking Latina, illiterate in both English and Spanish, becomes the vice president of her children's school advisory board on bilingual education. For some of these people who have not had the benefit of formal education and who have faced many challenges experienced by poor and working-class immigrants, it has been a struggle, a long road walked, a vision coming to realization.

Casa CHE is an innovative, clinic-based, community health education program that works directly with community residents to promote health and encourages residents to engage in actions designed to improve their living conditions and general well being. Initially formed to address mental-health issues in the Latino community, the model was later used to address many issues, including HIV. The approach has particular relevance for low-income, largely monolingual Spanish-speaking populations.

Each community has its own cultural context that affects the individuals who move within its boundaries. If the goal of health education is to make the community a healthier place in which to live and grow and to promote change, the health educator must also be able to work within the same cultural boundaries. As such, Casa CHE involved people from the community as health promoters who were trusted, understood the cultural context through experience, were role models, and were natural "communicators." The projects conducted under the auspices of Casa CHE drew from health education models used in Latin America and found that culturally relevant health education approaches are key to effective interventions that seek to address issues like HIV in the Latino community.

Casa CHE projects described in this chapter integrate popular health education theory and practice at a community clinic (La Clínica De La Raza) in Oakland, California. This chapter includes a description of the development of the components of a model of community health education; some of these components are still implemented today, while others have evolved into new projects.

This chapter begins with a description of the origin and evolution of Casa CHE projects, discusses relevent theory, addresses problems that arose, and concludes with lessons learned and criteria for projects to begin to be community driven. These criteria include training sessions that help community members go beyond individual lifestyle change to promoting changes that promote health in their environment. The skill-based trainings emphasize group development, popular health education, community diagnosis, and planning among other training elements. In addition, the projects should include a process whereby trainings result in an action to change the environment that is collectively designed and implemented by community members, and set up structures that permit ongoing praxis.

At the heart of the development of the Casa CHE projects is a position paper drafted in 1978 and entitled *Plan De Cinco Años* (Hernández, 1978), which set the foundation for the community health education and empowerment model that evolved into several distinct projects over a sixteen-year period. This health educator, Eberado Hernández, had been inspired by the work of Paulo Freire.

ORIGIN AND EVOLUTION OF CASA CHE PROJECTS

Casa En Casa

The original project called *Casa En Casa* (CEC) addressed the physical, mental, socioeconomic and environmental factors affecting the Latino community of East Oakland, California. Community health educators (CHEs) from La Clínica's community health education component (Casa CHE) went directly into the homes of neighborhood residents to facilitate health education sessions and to address issues of interest to the participants.

The first CEC groups were organized in 1979 in Oakland's Fruitvale district, which is comprised of largely low-income and working-class neighborhoods with ethnically diverse populations. Community health educators first recruited "hosts" for the meetings through mailings describing the project and its goals, person-to-person contact, and brief presentations to La Clínica patients. These persons then met with the CHE to plan the first meeting, agreed to host the meeting in their home, and recruited their neighbors and friends to attend.

Parents, residents, their families, friends, and neighbors came together at the block level with the goal of forming networks between neighborhoods that would grow incrementally. CEC meetings encouraged dialogue about health issues, discussion about La Clínica's services, provided education about these issues, and organized support for much needed health care. These meetings were conducted in Spanish.

Another goal, as stated in the original position paper, was to act in unison with community residents to promote health and to take action to improve living conditions and well-being. The encouragement of grassroots unity and leadership were among other goals. The idea was that every provision of service should also be a provision of organizing.

The strengths and skills that the hosts brought to the groups were many. Most of them had organized other family and community events and already had some leadership, organizing, and communication skills. They belonged to a variety of community and church organizations and came from a strong tradition of family and community values.

The hosts also experienced a myriad of barriers to organizing, including high mobility, lack of time for meetings, shortage of resources, and lack of child care. Immigrant populations living in the United States experience many levels of disenfranchisement. Not only may they be poor, but they may not speak English and are not afforded support systems available to other low-income people. People who participated in the project were typically already over-worked (many worked more than one job). Low turnout was common at meetings and conferences, since there were so many other demands in the people's personal lives.

Meeting in the home and neighborhood addressed some of the barriers to participation like safety, no child care, and lack of transportation. Sessions were held at times convenient to the participants (evenings and Saturdays), so that working women and men could attend. Refreshments were provided.

During the first meeting of each group, the project was described and a verbal assessment was done. Some meetings addressed health education issues, while others addressed social problems or concerns about the clinic. Topics covered included HIV education, infant care, nutrition, group dynamics, family planning, male involvement in family life, pregnancy and birth, parent and youth communication, and immigration rights. Discussions were shaped by a great concern about children.

Simultaneously, CEC groups were involved in various community actions, from mobilizing to oppose cutbacks in human services at the County Board of Supervisors to raising money to prevent cutbacks in child care. Letter-writing campaigns, testimonies to federal legislators, and meetings with state Assemblypersons about the importance of perinatal care took place. One group raised money for an annual scholarship for a local alternative school, Emiliano Zapata Street Academy, to be awarded to the graduating student who demonstrated outstanding scholastic achievement and community commitment. This group also opened a small credit union account for emergency needs. Other groups held meetings with local city councilpersons about violence in the schools and in the streets.

Two community *kermess* (street fairs) were organized in the early 1980s to "honor the community." A rare event in a high-crime area, the *kermess* drew 400 and 700 persons, respectively, had music and children's events, raised funds for family vendors, and addressed social issues affecting youth.

Documents from 1983 indicated that goals were constantly being redefined. The emphasis was on "the creation of consciousness in individuals and in the community; to build leadership; to form a coordinated network of CEC groups; to advocate for an informed community and to secure improved living conditions" (Hernández, 1983). These ideals also included collectivism, political action, and community involvement. As parents' and CHEs' skills developed, so did CEC. Hosts were involved in designing and implementing community conferences (see *intercambios* in the next section), and later on developed yearly health education plans.

The roles of the health educators and parents involved in the groups evolved. Hosts also became more involved in organizing and facilitating the meetings in their homes and, in one instance, a group met every other meeting without the participation of a health educator. The idea of the community organizer as someone involved in a long-term effort for the progressive transformation of the community was stressed. Genaro Vásquez Rojas, a Mexican educator and organizer, was shown with a sign saying, "The teacher who is organizing is also teaching." Not only were knowledge of and trust in the people prerequisites to community organizing, but optimism, mutual support, and commitment were important considerations.

Intercambios (Parent and Youth Conferences)

In 1982, the first of a series of biannual *intercambios* (conferences) was organized by the members from a particular CEC group who chose themes, facilitators, and activities; the members then coorganized and cofacilitated the actual conference. The goal was to bring together the various CEC groups around similar issues and concerns. The *intercambios* were held on Saturdays at local churches, and food and child care were provided. The *intercambio* themes were: "Communication with Our Children about Sex"; "Raising Our Children in the Environment in Which We Live"; "Know Your Rights!"; and "Improving the Health of Our Community." One conference featured youth from local schools and was entitled, "Oakland's Problems: A Youth's Point of View."

CHEs assisted with the production of a silk-screen poster for each event and mailing. Attendance varied from forty parents at one *intercambio* to 100 parents, who arrived in pouring rain, at another. It is estimated that 500 persons participated in CEC groups in the early years.

Promotores de la Salud (Health Promoters)

The concept of health promoters or *promotores de la salud* was integrated into the earlier activities. These were originally the hosts from previous years and served as parent peer educators. At one point, both the health educators and promoters voiced the need for improved coordination among the groups. The *comité central* (organizing committee) grew out of this. This group of promoters, with support from CHEs, began to plan activities for the project as a whole. They decided that each group should remain autonomous in planning activities and health education workshops, while the *comité* could represent the groups as a steering committee and develop yearly plans.

Yearly Plans: *Capacitaciones* (Trainings)

The first of the year-long plans was titled, "Plan '87." The organizing committee felt that promoter trainings (*capacitaciones*) should take place in a structured fashion to improve coordination among groups and so that promoters would have the same information. They decided that a yearly calendar of events, trainings, and conferences would be planned for the aforementioned purposes. One of the promoters helped produce a curriculum guide in Spanish for the first training.

Early promoter trainings were intended to be different from health education meetings, in that the trainings would stress both learning the material and learning how to teach it. This required planning agendas that covered the main points of the health education topic, addressed low literacy, and were culturally appropriate. The promoters were trained as cofacilitators and served as resource persons in their communities.

The first series, entitled *Aprendiendo a Enseñar: Hablando Con Los Hijos Acerca Del Sexo* (Learning to Teach: Talking with Our Children about Sex) took place on three consecutive Saturdays. Young parents and grandparents took part in activities on prevention of teen pregnancy, birth, values, reproductive systems, HIV, and others. The entire training was conducted in Spanish.

One grandparent, a monolingual elderly Mexican man, participated fully in the activities, including those that might be considered sensitive, like reproductive systems and birth. He commented that even though he was a little embarrassed at first, he felt that this was "natural" and that he wished he had known about these topics years before, when his wife was pregnant, so he could have helped more. The majority of the promoters, like this man, had an average third grade level of formal education. Similar comments were made by others, including a grandmother who felt so strongly about HIV prevention that she began to educate her children and grandchildren.

Plan '87 included sessions on first aid for children, accident prevention in the home, HIV/AIDS, control of diabetes and hypertension, stress, immigration rights, sexual assault prevention, and teen pregnancy prevention. One session focused entirely on learning techniques to facilitate the CEC sessions in the homes. It included theory and practice on how to lead discussions and set up activities.

As the La Clínica Board of Directors elections approached, the organizing committee coordinated participation in recruitment of the membership to promote representation on the Board for prevention activities for health. Subsequently, three CEC promoters were elected to the Board of Directors.

APPLICATION OF THEORY

A variety of theories in health education and other fields can be applied to development of projects at Casa CHE. Paulo Freire's work influenced the methods used (Freire, 1976). Health educators attended workshops with Paulo Freire and learned about popular education and the work of base communities in Latin American that had begun cooperatives there. A Brazilian educator, Freire developed ideas that have been applied in many parts of the world and in many fields, including health education. Included in his work are the ideas that no education is ever neutral, and as such, should be designed to be liberating; that education should start with the experience of the participants and should be relevant to their experience; that problem-posing and diaglogue-promoting activities should be used; that ongoing reflection and action (praxis) is key; and that individual and social transformation are goals. Education that addressed social justice issues was fundamental (Hope and Timmel, 1984).

During the first meetings of each CEC group, a verbal assessment was introduced, in broad terms, to promote a view of health that encompassed physical, mental, and socioeconomic aspects. Classes and meetings were planned to reflect the issues and topics stated by the parents. This was similar to the first step in Paulo Freire's codification process (Freire, 1973), where key issues and topics are identified. Health was the unifying theme. Since environmental issues and policy affect health, the groups met to discuss both health promotion and social issues. Mexican parents of small children requested workshops on the history of immigration laws, racism, the high school drop-out rate, HIV and AIDS, infant mortality in East Oakland, and substance abuse. One group mapped out the institutions and merchants in their neighborhood to identify resources and problem areas.

Substance abuse continued to be an area of concern to parents. Children of two groups played near areas where dirty needles, violence, and garbage were rampant. One group arranged a meeting with local youth who were vandalizing the neighborhood to find solutions and began approaching the city to clean up the streets. Another group met with a local school board member and local youth to find solutions to violence in the schools.

In another application of theory, David Reed's principles of education for building a people's movement were drawn upon, and included using the "social experience of the learners as the basic content, the raw material of the learning process" (Reed, 1981). Many of the CEC parents had completed only three years of formal education. They learned and based knowledge on their personal experiences and on the experiences of others. Dialogue and action-oriented activities (as opposed to lectures or reading) were based on the experience of the parents. Education was a valued resource. Groups held sessions on different health education topics. Survival English (English for a health crash course) provided one group the ability to call for an ambulance or get help in an emergency.

Social Support

Well-being is defined by cultural values, healing traditions, social structure, and the environment in which one lives. Family and community are strong cultural values and mechanisms for survival among Latinos. Studies carried out at the clinic had suggested a link between social isolation and negative pregnancy outcome. One Mexicana stated that stress (*nervios*) was caused by fear of letting her children out of the house. In her home town, all the children played outside for hours with little supervision because everyone knew each other.

For these reasons, CEC was held in the home. Various benefits resulted. Social support and a sense of community were nurtured among neighbors and family with similar concerns. Meeting in the home helped create an atmosphere of trust, so that sensitive issues around topics like HIV/AIDS could arise and be addressed. People eventually began to seek each other out as resources outside of group activities. The groups also served as organizing units.

People who did not typically participate in health education sessions, such as men, became involved in CEC. One example involved a family where the mother was the promotor of the CEC group held in their home. After three months of meetings, she arrived at the organizing committee meeting and tearfully told the group that her husband now participated in family activities. They have eight children, and both parents work. The father had spent previous holidays out with friends drinking, and the wife had threatened separation on numerous occasions. Through the CEC meetings, the father began to participate increasingly in discussions about family issues, teen pregnancy, communication, and the like. The mother related that after this he began spending more time interacting with the family and spent the entire holiday with them.

Natural Leaders

Promotores de la Salud (health promoters) were the peer parent educators, previously known as hosts, who invited neighbors and family members to their homes and cofacilitated meetings. They also served as resources in their communities and nutured the support networks. As Barbara Israel points out, the advantage of consistently identifying the person to whom others naturally turn for advice, emotional support, and tangible aid in the neighborhood (natural helper) is that that person, as *promotora,* already knows many of the issues and has organizational support (Israel, 1985).

These promotors were selected in various ways. Some were recommended by others in the community as trusted persons who could make a commitment and who were resource persons for others in the community. Others were persons who volunteered to organize groups in their home, and one promotor was a mother of five who could not attend groups outside her home (no child care).

Traditional community organizing theories were not as easily applied. For example, "The basic Alinsky approach emphasized organizing in the consumer mode by assembling preexisting organization into a kind of dense pack and propelling this . . . towards a visible local decision-making structure to force it to do what the neighborhood wanted" (McKnight and Kretzman, 1984). John McKnight and John Kretzman also point out in their article that "the neighborhood" has changed. Not only is there more mobility, causing the neighborhood's border and sense of community to become fuzzy, but the target in organizing is many times harder to define, much less to reach. These authors state that the three characteristics assumed necessary to effectively target the enemy (he or she is visible, local, and capable of resolving the problem) have changed (McKnight and Kretzman, 1984). Also, Saul Alinsky–style organizing emphasized the importance of an organizer getting in, organizing the community around an issue, and getting out so as not to create dependency. This may not always be appropriate, as the participatory process is more long term. Nina Wallerstein states, "Historically, . . . community organizing has differed from empowering education in its emphasis on winnable goals rather than on a participatory process that engages people in critical analysis of root causes as the basis for social action" (Wallerstein and Bernstein, 1988).

THE PROBLEMS

The Casa CHE projects accomplished a great deal; however, health educators continued to raise questions about the work. One of these had to do with the concept of the *promotora.* Even though promoters were perceived as taking a leadership role in designing yearly plans and organizing meetings in their homes, the health educators at Casa CHE continued to be primarily responsible for initiating and facilitating meetings, conferences, and actions. In essence, the question became, was this work community driven? Did the promoters choose, design, and implement the projects?

Returning to Paulo Freire (Freire, 1973, 1976) and the work outlined in *Helping Health Workers Learn* (Werner and Bower, 1982), *promotores* were expected to cofacilitate meetings. If empowerment was the goal, then some degree of independence from health educators was necessary. Training parents to educate and facilitate addressed criteria for activities that are community supportive rather than community oppressive (Werner, 1980). Yet, it appeared that skill-based trainings that prepared parents as educators were not enough. The unanswered question for us, as La Clínica health educators, was, When do we step out of a group? What skills will prepare the group to continue meeting by itself and investigate and design its own interventions, albeit with health educator support, not leadership? And was this a realistic expectation? As health educators, some of us had had years of experience and had practiced facilitating for lengthy periods of time before feeling comfortable as facilitators. Can we expect a parent to attend a series of trainings and then lead a group with little assistance?

Another problem arose from the fact that the support provided by the health educators was funded by various state, federal, and local grants. Restrictions tied to categorical funds limited the type of work that could be carried out and led to burnout and the need for creativity within the organization. General cutbacks during the Reagan years led to layoffs and the need to redirect staff energy. Each time something like this occurred, the consistency necessary for the project to grow and build upon itself suffered, participation lagged, and groups stopped meeting. This was another reason why models for encouraging self-sufficiency in the work were so important. Finally, this type of work was labor intensive and did not yield the kind of numbers that are found in traditional health education. For example, many of the HIV/AIDS contractors only allowed for a work plan that reached large numbers of persons with one-shot presentations. They would not fund projects that included a more comprehensive and critical analysis of underlying factors impacting on HIV/AIDS in the Latino community.

Another area where questions arose had to do with the focus of the education. While the philosophy and activities involved in these health education efforts included looking at social justice issues and organizing for social change, the actual health education workshops primarily focused on health topics (HIV, teen pregnancy prevention, hypertension, mental health) for individual lifestyle change. The promoters were prepared as peer educators and their message was primarily about learning ways to live healthier lives, change bad eating habits, communicate with their children, and so forth. This effort was important as part of the overall health education intervention. Yet a gap existed, whereby the promoters had not yet participated in systematic skill-based trainings that prepared them to analyze health issues and interventions, including organizing collective efforts that changed the environment in which they lived. Some of the theoretical questions around community organizing applied here.

Trainings tended to be based on knowledge or health content area. Discussions were held about how larger social issues contributed to these problems and the need to change the social environment to help solve the problems. Yet, models and tools for organizing to change these factor remained as gaps. Subsequently, groups organized around social issues and focused on lifestyle change. In essence, health education workshops about specific content areas lent themselves to individual behavior changes as the focus for community members.

The importance of this point is demonstrated through the work of H. L. Blum (1981), who segregates factors affecting health into four groupings: (1) medical care services, (2) lifestyle, (3) heredity, and (4) environment (physical, natural and man-made, sociocultural, economic, education, employment, and so forth). The author states that these four groupings "lend themselves to the analytic and synthesizing tasks facing anyone who desires to plan for better health." He goes on to describe "the relative importance of the four aggregates of forces that have the major effects on health. . . . Clearly, the largest aggregate of forces resides in the person's environment. One's own behavior, in great part derived from one's experience with one's environment, is seen as the next largest force affecting health. Medical care services have been segregated out from the environment because of our great interest and investment in them. They make a modest contribution to health status" (Blum, 1981). The author goes on to say that heredity is a lesser force.

Participating in CEC and the organizing committee raised the awareness of many of the promoters about the difference between access to medical care (in the clinic) and the promotion of community health. Members of CEC began to be aware of the importance of addressing environmental and social issues, and of health education for environmental change so that families and communities could live in a health-promoting environment.

THE NEXT STAGE: TOWARD HEALTH EDUCATION FOR ENVIRONMENTAL CHANGE

The Application of Popular Health Education

In 1988 and 1989, some of the community health educators traveled to Guadalajara, Mexico, and were able to work with public-health students as they applied popular health education principles

there. They watched as public-health students worked with marginalized communities. In one instance, the members of a community
identified gastrointestinal disorders as one of their primary health
issues. Community members designed and implemented a community diagnosis that included going door to door to ask questions
about water acquisition and use. Community members (many of
whom could not read or write) collected and analyzed the data and
concluded that the lack of potable water was the problem. They then
organized and got relief from local authorities. Health education
students provided support for community members, who did everything from design the assessment tool, implement the survey,
design educational materials, come up with a slate of environmental solutions, and organize themselves and acquire what they
needed—from proper drainage systems to paved streets—so that
water trucks could bring potable water. At each step of the process,
the health educators only provided assistance, and used techniques
such as asking critical questions to help promoters in the process of
designing their projects. Providing peer education and designing
educational materials about healthy habits was part of this effort.

The clinic's health educators also learned about a *manzana* model
used in Mexico, in which each block area within a certain region of
a primary clinic was considered a *manzana* and was assigned a promoter from the community. The promoter would implement health
education campaigns with community members who lived there.

When the clinic's health educators returned to the United States,
they shared what they had learned with their fellow health educators. Lengthy discussions ensued about how the work that was described in Mexico could be applied to conditions affecting the East
Oakland Latino community. Another question had to do with the
application of popular health education principles in the United
States. A gradual shift led to the development of projects that went
beyond a focus on education for individual lifestyle change to
projects that also looked at community-level change solutions. This
orientation was written into funding proposal work plans.

The grant work plan was written so that *promotores* would be
recruited and trained about both lifestyle and environmental factors impacting on the health issue. These promoters would then
conduct a community diagnosis of the health issue and collectively
plan and implement an action that would change the environment.

As such, in 1989, a hypertension project involved recruiting and
training indigenous promoters about both lifestyle and socioeconomic factors that contribute to high rates of hypertension in the
Latino community. Promoters were required to diagnose the problem
in their community and choose an action that they could collectively work on and that would, in some way, change the environ-

ment in which they live with respect to hypertension. In this case, the promoters identified the problem of lack of access to quality low-cost nutrition in the inner cities as a contributing social factor to high rates of hypertension. Over a period of two years, these primarily Spanish-speaking promoters conducted a feasibility study (with local university students), sold low-cost produce on Saturdays to members and others, began a food cooperative with a board of directors and membership fees, and sought grant funding for a permanent food cooperative. They also conducted peer education in the community about lifestyle factors contributing to hypertension.

In a similar effort at the same time, a tobacco control grant was designed so that youth and adult promoters were recruited and trained to provide peer education, diagnose the problem of tobacco access and promotion in their community, and implement community-level solutions. In this case, they implemented a "purchase survey" of where underage youth bought cigarettes, publicized the results (90% success rate), and carried out a merchant education campaign to reduce sales to minors. This was markedly different from more traditional health education efforts that focused solely on lifestyle factors to improve health.

In 1991, a health educator conducted interviews with the promoters who had been with Casa CHE for a number of years and assessed their strengths, needs, and perceptions regarding their roles in the projects. The assessment revealed that the promoters knew that they were seen as leaders, but felt they lacked the tools to truly do this. They also questioned the difference between a promoter and a CHEista and their respective roles. Out of this grew the idea for the *Escuela Para Promotores* (school for promoters).

The *escuela* was a ten-session course that was held every six months to train promoters in health education skills. Promoters interested in participating completed a brief application and made a commitment to attend all ten sessions. The sessions were interactive and focused on skill building. In the first session, promoters defined the role of a promoter, entered into games that fostered dialogue about community health education work, and set personal skill and knowledge-based goals for themselves. Following sessions focused on group process skills (how to run groups), facilitation skills for educational workshops and organizing meetings, decision-making skills and models, popular education skills and techniques, learning skills to analyze health issues and design interventions to change the environment, basic elements for planning events, designing a yearly plan, and conducting evaluations.

For example, in the session on health analysis, the promoters were given a list of health issues and problems. The four factors affecting health were described (Blum, 1981). The promoters were asked to choose which of the four factors would primarily impact on their health issue and explain why they had chosen it. A discussion ensued about the reason why the environment in which one lives most affects health. Promoters were then asked to work in small groups to design programs that would promote environmental-change solutions for the health issues they had discussed.

After the sessions were completed, promoters who had attended all ten sessions graduated and received diplomas. The last sessions were devoted to planning and evaluating a specific action that this group of promoters had chosen. As such, the role of the promoter developed from a cofacilitator or peer educator to a designer of community-health actions and programs. To date, four *escuelas* have been conducted. Each graduated a class of ten to fifteen health promoters. Every class organized an event or action that would impact the health of the community. By the end of the last two *escuelas*, it became evident that the promoters had not yet formed an entity separate from the CHEs. Tensions and frustrations began to grow within the promoters. A meeting was held, where the promoters developed a list of concerns and suggested a plan of action. The plan is currently underway and is being evaluated at regular intervals. This process is spearheaded by promoters with limited participation of CHEs.

In a sense, this situation was a test to see if promoters would organize themselves, how they would confront an issue, what structures they would develop, and what the process would be like. It took a small crisis to unite the group, and community leaders emerged with increased support and decreased intervention from the CHEs; the promoters had passed the test.

Promoters now have monthly meetings where they are responsible for facilitation, setting the agenda, evaluating the session, follow-up, and action. Structures and systems are being developed at every meeting to bridge communication gaps, set rules, and define their roles as promoters and their relationship to CHE and the clinic. The challenge for CHEs was to step back and provide technical assistance and support, but to limit actual intervention. The promoters needed to take responsibility for the well-being of their groups and search for solutions to their groups' problems and obstacles. This process brought with it a cohesion that had not previously existed.

Promoters continue to face challenges, including funding structures, the structure of the clinic and Casa CHE, and their own life needs. They are involved in their school PTAs and Bilingual Education Boards. Several new CEC groups have emerged, with promoters leading each session, and local schools are benefiting in their

HIV/AIDS programs, where promoters serve as educators in the classrooms. They have organized awareness campaigns around state propositions and political candidates, are involved in voter registration drives, and have started to plan post-election activities.

Finally, as the first *escuela* was being designed, it became evident that the fifteen CHEs (two of whom were previous health promoters) had not dialogued about what was meant by popular education, empowerment, health education, and the like. Staff trainings were conducted that covered everything from popular education theory, techniques, and models; techniques that promote dialogue, critical thinking, and use critical questions; and how to balance lifestyle and environmental change solutions.

In summary, the early trainings—*capacitaciones*—developed into skill-based trainings in the form of the *escuela* to prepare health promoters as health educators. *Capacitaciones* that are health-content-area-based continued on and addressed a variety of health issues in the community. The CEC neighborhood meetings became an arena for the promoters who had graduated from the *escuela* to go out into the community, teach others, and organize actions. Finally, grants were written reflecting this new model.

Unfortunately, some contracts which could appropriately apply the models described previously (such as in HIV/AIDS prevention) have only recently begun to allow interventions that went beyond one-shot educational presentations (that may reach large numbers of people), to those that look at underlying factors and environmental change approaches.

CONCLUSION

Health educators have found that, for projects to begin to be community driven and self-sufficient, at least four criteria must be met:

1. That trainings go beyond addressing lifestyle and individual behavior-change models to include models that help community members change the place where they live so that it promotes health and healthy behaviors.

2. That indigenous health-promoter trainings be skill based, and go beyond health-content areas and peer education to focus on skills that develop groups and include health education and other competencies (such as community diagnosis and organizing, planning, evaluation, health-issue analysis and interventions to change the environment, and many more).

3. That projects are written to move promoters through training and diagnosis of a health issue, and that this result in at least

one actual action that trainees have collectively investigated, planned, and will implement and evaluate to improve their environment. This action must address a specific health issue and must change the environment to promote health.

4. That structures are integrated that allow for ongoing praxis by promoters of the skills they have learned.

Finally, the model devised for grant work plans integrated these ideas and included the following activities: *Promotores* would be recruited and trained about both lifestyle and environmental factors impacting on the health issue. These promoters would then conduct a community diagnosis of the health issue and collectively plan and implement an action that would change the environment. By undertaking this comprehensive approach, health educators can go beyond one-shot HIV/AIDS education to a model that stresses structural and long-term changes—both in the individuals who receive the education and the community as a whole.

NOTE

In recognition of the promoters and health educators at Casa CHE for their long-term commitment to the community. Special thanks to Eberado S. Hernández for many years of dedication to building Casa CHE and to Mele Smith for her insightful comments.

REFERENCES

Blum, H. L., (1981). *Planning for Health.* New York: Human Services Press.
Freire, Paulo. (1973). *Education and Conscientizacao* (Education for Critical Consciousness). New York: Seabury Press.
Freire, Paulo. (1976). Pedagogy of the Oppressed (summary). In *The Planning of Change,* edited by W. G. Bennis et al. 3d ed. New York: Holt, Rinehart & Winston.
Hernández, Eberardo S. (1978). *Plan De Cinco Años.* Oakland, Calif.: La Clínica De La Raza.
Hernández, Eberardo S. (1983). *Considerations for Community Organizers.* Oakland, Calif.: La Clínica De La Raza.
Hope, Ann, and Sally Timmel. (1984). *Training for Transformation.* Gweru, Zimbabwe: Mambo Press.
Israel, B. A. (1985). Social Networks and Social Support: Implications for Natural Helper and Community Level Interventions. *Health Education Quarterly* 12(1): 65–80.
McKnight, J., and J. Kretzman. (1984). Community Organizing in the 80's: Toward a Post-Alinsky Agenda. *Social Policy* 14: 15–17.
Reed, D. (1981). Social Education. In *Education for Building a People's Movement.* Boston: South End Press.

Wallerstein, Nina, and Edward Bernstein. (1988). Empowerment Education: Freire's Ideas Adapted to Health Education. *Health Education Quarterly* 15(4): 379–394.

Werner, David. (1980). Health Care & Human Dignity: A Subjective Look at Community-Based Rural Health Programs in Latin America. *Contact,* Special Series 3: 91–95.

Werner, David, and Bill Bower. (1982). *Helping Health Workers Learn.* Palo Alto, Calif.: The Hesperian Foundation.

8

HIV Prevention Strategies with Homeless and Street Youth

*Meredith Larson and
Melissa Schatz*

Each week, new youth are added to the flow of young people living on the streets of San Francisco, part of the estimated 1.5 million homeless adolescents nationwide. They flee their homes to escape physical violence, sexual abuse, emotional abuse, or other family problems. They may also leave because of economic hardship or to escape difficulties in their school or community; sometimes because of discrimination based on their sexual preference, race, or other sociodemographic characteristics. Other homeless young people are known as "throwaways," forced to leave their homes because their parents either do not want or can not handle the youth, or because they cannot financially support them.

Youth often survive on the streets by panhandling, stealing, selling drugs, or exchanging sex for money, food, rides, drugs, or a place to sleep. Some runaway and homeless adolescents access services on a regular basis; others intermittently, if at all. To escape the pain, many of these young people turn to drugs and alcohol. A San Francisco Department of Public Health study published in August 1993 showed that "30% of Larkin Street youth are injection drug users (IDU)." Often, injection drug–using youth share their syringes, placing themselves at great risk for contracting HIV. The same study also showed that "more than 30% engage in sex with IDUs and 25% have received money or drugs for sex." Of the young men surveyed, "16.6% engage in same sex behaviors and 17.2% engage in sex with males and females" (Bermudez and Shalwitz, 1993:3). For many reasons, youth in this population may not practice safer sex with either sexual partners or prostitution clients.

The severity of this situation reflects itself in the HIV seroprevalence among Larkin Street clients. The same 1993 SFDPH study of 308 youth using the Larkin Street Youth Center Clinic showed that 9.3 percent are HIV positive (Bermudez and Shalwitz, 1993:3). In the larger homeless youth population, a 1990 study of 4,383 runaway and homeless youth in four states found 4.13 percent to be HIV infected.

AGENCY DESCRIPTION

Larkin Street Youth Center (LSYC) provides services to approximately 1,000 homeless and runaway young people each year. Larkin Street Youth Center's mission is to "create a network of communities that inspire youth to move beyond the streets, [nurturing] potential, [promoting] dignity, and [supporting] bold steps by all." A nonprofit, community-based agency, Larkin first opened its doors in 1984.

The agency provides a continuum of care services for youth. These services include a Drop-In Center for twelve to seventeen year olds, Case Management, an Aftercare program for eighteen to twenty-three year olds, a street-based Outreach program, and a residential component which provides emergency overnight shelter and foster placement. In conjunction with the San Francisco Department of Public Health and the San Francisco Unified School District, LSYC is able to provide a free clinic for its clients and an education program in the Drop-In Center. LSYC also has a business component to provide job opportunities and job training for youth. The business component is in the process of opening a Ben & Jerry's "partnershop," an ice cream shop that will employ street youth.

Through these services, Larkin works with a diverse population of homeless youth. Most youth are from outside of San Francisco, and in fiscal year 1993, 16 percent were from other countries. Clients are of varied ethnicities and sexualities, and a significant per-centage are monolingual Spanish-speaking youth. In Case Management, 75 percent of clients reported having a history of child abuse and 46 percent reported a history of attempted suicide.

LSYC has been involved with HIV prevention since opening ten years ago, conducting such work through the continuum of services at the agency. In this chapter, we focus on prevention education and services offered by the Outreach and Drop-In departments. Outside of these areas, case managers provide intensive one-on-one HIV education and counseling, as well as HIV pre- and post-test counseling. LSYC has also developed a comprehensive plan for on-site HIV testing and treatment services for youth who are HIV infected. HIV testing is conducted by the LSYC clinic, and treatment plans are designed by an HIV Clinical Team. The Aftercare program primarily serves eighteen to twenty-three year olds who are HIV positive, providing case management services, housing, and food.

BARRIERS TO PREVENTION

As HIV prevention educators working with runaway and homeless youth, our goal is to provide education that is accessible and which promotes behavior change. In order to accomplish this goal, we need to understand and address the barriers that are intrinsic to our task. These barriers not only center around our ability to access and engage this population, but also center around the barriers to HIV prevention behavior faced by homeless youth. Getting past these barriers requires spontaneity, perseverance, and an understanding of issues facing homeless young people.

The first barrier we encounter in prevention education is gaining access to the homeless and street youth population, as they are often a hidden population. To find homeless youth, the LSYC Outreach team literally walks the streets in areas where homeless youth congregate, as well as networks with other agencies that may have contact with these youth. Once we do gain access to them, we must address the mistrust of adults and service providers that this population often feels. In our first contact with a youth, our goal is to begin establishing a trusting relationship and a comfortable rapport; such a relationship is the foundation to the effectiveness of our intervention. Prevention educators may also have restricted time with youth due to the transient nature of the homeless youth population. Clients may move on within a short time; to go back home, into placement, or to a different city or state. Even if a youth makes regular contact with the center, prevention educators may find themselves pitted against the appeal of the streets.

Prior to contact with Larkin, homeless young people often lack adequate information on how to prevent HIV infection and, many times, lack access to condoms, bleach, and HIV testing services. Unfortunately, even if these youth have adequate HIV prevention education, they may not practice HIV prevention behavior. The reasons behind their unsafe behavior can be varied and complex.

The emotional issues facing Larkin clients, such as low self-esteem, history of abuse, and "passive suicidality," present one of the largest barriers to HIV prevention behavior. These young people may feel a sense of powerlessness in relationships, neediness, self-destructiveness, or suicidal feelings. Not only do many of these youth feel a lack of control over what happens to their bodies, but they also lack skills to negotiate safer sex or safe needle usage. In expression of passive suicidality, some homeless youth may not care whether they live, or may even wish themselves to be dead, and therefore not take action to prevent HIV infection. A youth with a history of sexual abuse, which is the case with many homeless teens, may experience significant shame and powerlessness about their sexuality and their bodies. Embarrassment and shame around sexuality presents a barrier to HIV prevention behavior. Though homeless youth may be sexually active, they may not feel comfortable with their own bodies, their sexuality, discussing sex, or engaging in safer-sex behaviors.

Activities associated with street survival also present a barrier to HIV prevention behavior. Involvement in survival sex, for example, increases a youth's risk for exposure to HIV; and, in addition to increased risk through multiple partners, youth often receive additional money in exchange for unprotected sex. Substance abuse, as well, may become a survival tool that increases HIV risk behavior. If they are using intravenously, youth are often in a situation where sharing a syringe is the only way they are going to get their "fix."

Because street youth are forced to focus so much of their thinking on their day-to-day survival needs, they often fail to recognize that their present behavior can have tragic consequences for their future well-being. The concept of a disease that can take ten or more years to manifest itself in illness becomes meaningless to young people who are having difficulty with day-to-day survival. Also, these adolescents often feel invincible in the face of risk—"it won't happen to me"—or that, if they do get into trouble, someone will rescue them. Denial around risk for HIV can be compounded by the fact that, although many young people are living with HIV, the people youth see dying from AIDS are in their twenties, thirties, or older, and hence do not view the disease as an issue for their age group.

A major barrier faced by HIV prevention educators at LSYC is to effectively reach all clients in a multicultural and multilingual environment. Prevention programs need to target various cultures, ethnicities, genders, sexualities, class backgrounds, and languages. Youth may also not be literate, or they may have limited English language skills. In addition, Larkin serves a number of immigrant youth, predominantly from Mexico and Central America, where they usually have had minimal, if any, access to HIV education.

A significant percentage of homeless and runaway youth are gay, lesbian, or bisexual. Many of these young people have been forced out of their homes because of their sexual orientation, or have run away from home because of homophobia within their families or communities. While they may have come to San Francisco to come out of the closet, gay youth may experience internalized homophobia. They may be in denial about their own sexual behavior and, consequently, their risk for HIV. Also, a gay or bisexual youth may feel that he deserves to contract HIV, believing it is a gay men's disease and therefore a judgment on his sexual orientation. Young gay or bisexual men may also feel, with such high HIV seroprevalence in the gay community, that they are doomed to contract HIV no matter what they do. Young lesbian women may believe that they are not at risk for HIV because of the myth that "lesbians don't get HIV," no matter what risk behaviors they engage in.

STREET-BASED OUTREACH HIV PREVENTION EDUCATION

The purpose of LSYC's street-based Outreach HIV prevention education is to affect knowledge, attitude, intention, and behavior. This program strives to (1) increase knowledge about HIV and AIDS, (2) change attitudes about HIV and associated risks, (3) promote intention to avoid high-risk activities, and (4) alter behavior accordingly. Outreach prevention work can be divided into three approaches: one-on-one, spontaneous groups, and formal groups. Sometimes one approach can lead to another. No matter how many people you are working with, the dynamics of the interaction will be affected by the street atmosphere. LSYC Outreach workers try to weed out those who are not in our target group. One way to do this is by carefully choosing where to interact with youth. Ideally, we want to isolate our target population from the rest of the street scene as much as possible during an intervention.

One-on-One Intervention

One-on-one intervention is the most frequent. Larkin Street Outreach workers use two tools to create an HIV prevention education interaction on the street. One tool is to distribute free condoms and bleach. By offering specific prevention supplies, we create an opportunity for a conversation around HIV prevention. The other tool is to offer free candy in exchange for answering an HIV question. We have found this to be one of the most effective techniques for creating a discussion around HIV prevention.

As we get to know what a youth's barriers to HIV prevention may be—their issues of survival (i.e., hustling, injection drug use, multiple sex partners)—we focus our intervention toward these areas. Outreach workers ask questions that give a sense of the client's baseline HIV knowledge and let the questions grow from there. Particularly with first interactions, we start with basic HIV questions. We have also found that, by asking questions that solicit the youth's opinions, we gain greater insight into their emotional barriers and, therefore, we can better address these issues. Occasionally, a long-time street client may have repeatedly answered all our best HIV questions. In these cases, we have them ask us a question; they must discuss the answer with us to earn their candy.

As street-based Outreach workers, we serve as a reminder to young people that they should protect themselves from HIV that evening. We are the reminder for them to carry condoms or to go to the needle exchange before it closes at 8 P.M. With clients who have expressed a desire to protect themselves from HIV but often forget to carry condoms or their own syringe, we have found it effective to offer these youth candy for showing us a condom from their pocket or, if applicable, their own syringe. When clients tell us how they protected themselves from HIV or taught a friend about HIV prevention, we also reward them with candy.

Spontaneous Street Groups

Spontaneous street groups occur when an Outreach worker gathers a group of young people for a quick HIV prevention discussion. This sometimes happens when a group of clients hear us ask someone a question. Another youth may jump in with questions of their own, instigated by the answer they overheard. Soon, we have a group of young people around us asking and answering questions for candy. Sometimes we have them quiz each other, or have them answer a more difficult question working together as a group.

Formal Street Groups

Formal street groups are planned events, which take more preparation and equipment. For formal street groups, LSYC Outreach uses a van, a VCR, an HIV prevention video, a table with literature, cookies and punch, and little prizes that can be distributed (such as condom key chains, socks, tee-shirts, or candy bars). Outreach workers comb the surrounding area to invite young people to the group. If the group can meet consistently in the same area one evening a week, it affects attendance positively. The VCR is set up next to the van, using an electrical adapter. A display table with condoms and literature is set up near the van as well. While the video is playing, Outreach workers serve cookies and punch to those who are watching the video. The Outreach worker facilitating the group periodically stops the video and asks the group HIV questions related to the information given in the video. Each person who answers a question is given a prize.

Helpful Tips for Street Outreach HIV Prevention Education

- Be relaxed, approachable, sex positive, and comfortable with HIV education.
- Be nonjudgmental and respectful.
- Get to know clients' names and get them to know your name.
- Use humor whenever possible. It relaxes you and the client.
- Use the youth's "language" as much as possible without being patronizing.
- Know what you are talking about.
- Keep condoms out in the open—in your hand or on the display table. Do not keep them a secret.
- Get as much information exchanged as possible during each interaction with a youth.
- If you are talking about condoms and latex barriers (for oral sex, mouth to vagina or anus), demonstrate their use. For example, if you are talking about how to make a latex barrier from a condom, take out a condom and show the youth how to make one from a nonlubed condom. If you are talking about how to put a condom on correctly, demonstrate on your Outreach partner's hand. If you are talking about HIV protection and oral sex, have the client take a nonlubed condom out of the package and taste it.
- Whether a youth is "out" or not, always include heterosexual and homosexual behaviors in presenting HIV prevention information.
- When new youth witness how "cool" you are with clients you know (i.e., nonjudgmental, informative, respectful, trustworthy), they will begin to trust you, too.
- When you answer a question, explain the answer as well as possible.

Examples of "Candy Questions"

Q: What are the three bodily fluids that transmit HIV?

A: Blood, semen, vaginal fluids.

Q: What is the difference between HIV and AIDS?

A: HIV is the virus that can cause AIDS. You can be HIV positive and not have AIDS. AIDS is when your immune system cannot fight off "opportunistic infections" that our bodies usually fight off all the time with no problem.

Q: How do you know if someone is HIV positive?

A: You can't tell by looking at someone or even by asking them. Not all people with HIV are sickly and not all sickly people have HIV.

Q: How does a person know if they are infected with HIV?

A: The only way you can tell is by getting an HIV antibody test. Sometimes if a person gets an infection common to persons with AIDS that may indicate they are HIV positive, but only an HIV antibody test will say for sure.

Q: How can you get HIV?

A: HIV has to enter your body when an infected person's blood, semen, or vaginal fluids enter your bloodstream through an open cut or sore. It only has to be a small cut, like tearing that happens to the mucous membrane in the vagina or anus during intercourse, or by sticking a dirty syringe in your body. You could also have small cuts or sores in your mouth or on your hands.

Q: What are eight reasons a condom might break?

A: Air in the condom, no reservoir tip, not enough lube, oil-based lube, "double bagging" (using two condoms at a time), tearing the condom with fingernails or teeth, condom is expired, condom is stored incorrectly (heat dries it out), condom is too small, genital piercing, and so on.

Q: What are ten ways you can have sex with someone that is safer than unprotected intercourse?

A: Use a condom, oral sex with a condom, oral sex and not swallowing ejaculate, mutual masturbation, masturbation in front of partner, rubbing bodies together, making out, talking about sex (as in fantasizing), phone sex, and so forth. (Educator explains different levels of risk for each activity.)

HIV PREVENTION EDUCATION IN THE DROP-IN CENTER

As with Outreach, staff in the Drop-In Center use a variety of strategies with young people to try to effect positive change in areas of knowledge, attitude, intention, and behavior. Once basic trust is established with the youth, staff can move on to basic HIV prevention education—through one-on-one interventions, groups, and having information and prevention supplies available. In addition, we strive to provide at least one one-on-one HIV prevention education session with every Drop-In Center client; all clients are asked to fill out an HIV education questionnaire as part of their Drop-In Center intake form. We use this worksheet as an introductory HIV education tool with clients, and with it we explain where condoms, bleach, and needle exchange cards are located; what HIV testing services are available for clients at the Larkin clinic; and what confidentiality laws protect the client if they are HIV positive. At the Center, we have two to three groups a week that directly relate to HIV prevention. These are run by the Drop-In HIV prevention specialist or educators from agencies Larkin collaborates with.

We have found two of the largest barriers to HIV prevention to be low self-esteem and passive suicidality. Strategies for breaking down these barriers may not even involve mentioning HIV, but rather involve attention and nurturing given to clients, support and encouragement, and helping them become involved in fun or meaningful activities intended to give their lives more joy or purpose. For example, our larger Drop-In HIV prevention program includes field trips to the beach, "Jurassic Park," a Native-American pow wow, the Lesbian and Gay Film Festival, and Cinco de Mayo festivities.

As part of delivering services to a multicultural population, our HIV prevention program must validate and support youth in their identities or cultures—ethnicity, nationality, sexuality, gender, class, and so on—and provide prevention education that is culturally relevant and culturally sensitive. At Larkin, close to 20 percent of the clients we serve are monolingual Latino youth; thus, it is very important that our services be bilingual as well as culturally sensitive to this population. Further, in addressing sexuality in HIV prevention work, educators are careful not to make assumptions regarding a youth's sexual preference or behaviors; and, consequently, not targeting interventions to certain sexual acts based on these assumptions.

An HIV prevention program with homeless youth must also be sensitive and supportive to those who already know that they are HIV positive or who may strongly believe that they are HIV positive. Though we as educators may want to bring home the realities of AIDS to youth, some scare tactics and comments such as "you wouldn't want to end up like this, would you?" may be hurtful to HIV positive youth and increase their depression around pending health problems or death. It is important in an HIV prevention program to also include discussions regarding prevention around reinfection.

HIV Prevention Groups and Activities

The Drop-In Center has an "HIV Prevention Activity Plan" form that helps us think strategically in terms of which barriers we want the activity to target and which populations of youth we want to reach. On the form, we have a section for focus objectives, such as reduce denial around risk, improve self-esteem, and increase healthy attitude toward sexuality. We have other sections for target population, name of activity, materials needed, preparation needed, and how activity is conducted.

Larkin staff have likened conducting groups in the Drop-In Center to "guerrilla education." In Drop-In, clients can come and go when they please; if what they see does not please them, they leave. Educational activities need to be flexible, engaging, and, when appropriate, entertaining. Groups should also be as participatory as possible; this allows young people to educate each other and share information and experiences, which improves self-esteem.

We have found it important to incorporate youth as peer educators whenever possible. Adolescents often turn to peers rather than adults for information on sex and drugs; thus, incorporating young people into an HIV prevention program on a formal or an informal basis is helpful in promoting safe behaviors among the target population. Further, through helping others and sharing their knowledge, adolescents may increase their self-esteem and begin to practice and maintain safe behaviors themselves. Clients can be incorporated as peer educators by assisting with groups, helping design intervention programming, showing other clients how to use condoms, doing informal outreach, and distributing information on Youth Needle Exchange.

In the following pages, we describe the activities listed below that are part of the LSYC model for the HIV prevention program in the Drop-In Center:

- Reproductive Anatomy and Sexuality
- Condom Demonstrations, Condom Relays, and Erotic Uses for Latex
- Sexual Decision Making
- Negotiation Skills
- Field Trips
- Wedge Program
- Art and HIV
- "Condom Sense" and Other Games
- Videos
- One-on-One Interventions
- Interventions around Injection Drug Use

Reproductive Anatomy and Sexuality We have found that many adolescents have not had access to basic information on reproduction, sexuality, and their own bodies. Having this knowledge can help give young people a sense of control over their own bodies and decrease embarrassment around sex and sexuality.

We have found that liveliness and humor work well with this activity. For this exercise, we use a flip chart with diagrams of reproductive systems and external genitalia. Pointing to diagrams of male and female reproductive anatomy, we ask participants to name body parts from the vas deferens to the Fallopian tubes and beyond. We discuss the women's reproductive cycle, menstruation, as well as the clitoris and its role in women's sexual pleasure. Using the male reproductive diagram, we explain the physiology of erection, and why "withdrawal" does not work to prevent pregnancy or STDs. The charts are used to launch into larger discussions of reproduction, sexuality, and sexual pleasure. We also recently acquired the Vulva Puppet, an anatomically correct puppet made of red and purple velvet and gold satin. The puppet has become a popular tool for these groups.

Condom Demonstrations, Condom Relays, and Erotic Uses for Latex We keep a penis model and condoms on hand for staff and volunteers to provide condom demonstrations for clients whenever possible. The more condom demonstrations done with youth—participating as well as watching—the more comfortable and knowledgeable they become with proper condom use.

When discussing problems with condom use, youth will often say that condoms break on them. We find this problem is usually because of incorrect usage. Therefore, we continually review the various steps regarding proper condom usage. Clients also cite lack of pleasure from latex and loss of erection as reasons why condoms do not work for them. In response, we educate them to approach condom use as part of sex play, as a sex toy, so that erections and sexual stimulation will not be as diminished. For example, a sexual partner can put the condom on the other partner as part of sex play; and keeping the condom nearby, open and ready, can minimize breaking the momentum. In addition, we discuss the use of water-based lubricants in increasing sexual pleasure.

If clients are interested, we teach them how to put condoms on with their mouth. This skill is important for those who engage in hustling or prostitution, as many prostitution clients request blow jobs but resist condom use. The technique for demonstrations is as follows: Place a non-lubricated condom in your mouth with the tip facing a cheek; use the mouth and tongue to then flip the condom so the tip is facing the roof of the mouth; using the mouth and tongue, position the condom over a penis model or two fingers closed together, and roll the condom down using the lips rather than the teeth. Usually, saliva from the mouth will "pinch the tip" so there will not be air bubbles, but one should always check to make sure there are no air bubbles.

We also show clients how to make latex barriers from non-lubed condoms for use with vaginal oral sex or rimming (mouth to anus). These barriers can be made by cutting off the tip of a condom (and the rim) with scissors or teeth and then cutting up the side—unroll and you have a square of latex.

Our experience indicates that many young people do not initially know that they should only use water-based lubricants with condoms. To visually demonstrate the importance of using only water-based lubricants, we blow up a condom into a balloon and rub baby oil or petroleum jelly (Vaseline) vigorously on the latex— the condom usually pops within thirty seconds.

Another popular activity is the Condom Relay. For this activity, two penis models are set up at the end of the room and the clients are lined up in two lines at the other end of the room (making sure the running or walking path is clear). Each youth is given a condom and is allowed to have the package open and ready. The participants are given instructions for the relay, which include reiterating the proper way to unroll a condom. When the signal is given, those at the front of the line run and unroll their condoms on the penis models while staff at each model watch to make sure it is done correctly. Then the youth takes the condom off, runs back to the line, and tags the next person, until each person in the line has a turn. The line that finishes first wins the game.

Sexual Decision Making   This activity allows young people to think through reasons why to choose to have sex and why to choose not to. The exercise supports positive decision making around sexuality and being in control over one's own body.

Using a chalkboard or flip chart, the facilitator writes at the top "why youth decide yes" and "why youth decide no." Then the facilitator engages participants in brainstorming reasons, first under the "yes" heading and then under the "no" heading. For "yes," clients might list the following: for fun, peer pressure, in love, to be macho or cool, rebellion, to have a kid, afraid their partner will leave, sex for money, and the like. "No" responses might be, do not feel ready or are scared, want to wait till in love or married, church, parents, reputation, pregnancy, STDs and HIV, and the like.

The facilitator makes sure issues of sexual abuse, rape, and survival sex (hustling) are acknowledged in this activity, pointing out that some young people may be sexually active but not due to their own choice. The facilitator includes in this discussion a person's right to his or her own body, stating that no one has the right to touch them or be sexual with them without their permission. The facilitator ensures that clients know of resources for support within the agency if a youth wants to discuss a current or past experience of abuse, and also lets the participants know that staff are open to further discussion of this issue after the group.

After the lists are created, the facilitator refers back to the "yes" list and asks the group, "Which of these reasons do you think are good reasons?" Then, the group does the same with the "no" list. From our experience, adolescents tend to strongly support only a few of the "yes" reasons as valid; adolescents tend to support most of the "no" reasons as valid. This exercise is intended to increase and support good decision-making skills, particularly around saying "no" when pressured to be sexually active. The facilitator points out that one may have chosen at one time to be sexually active, but may choose differently at other times.

Negotiation Skills There are different activities that we use to help young people develop negotiation skills. One such activity is safer-sex role plays. The facilitator brainstorms with the group to create two lists: "Why men don't use condoms" and "Why women don't use condoms." Answers for the men have included the following: don't like the way condoms feel, don't have a condom at the time, can't afford or can't get condoms, too drunk or high, embarrassed, denial of risk, love, and ego. For the women, answers have included, don't like the way condoms feel, afraid of rejection, afraid of angering partner, want to get pregnant, love, too drunk or high, and rape. The facilitator goes over the lists with the group, pointing out differences and similarities. Then the facilitator has participants verbally role play several of the situations, with one youth playing the part of the partner who wants to use a condom, another youth playing the part of the partner who doesn't want to use a condom, and another youth playing the part of the "helper" who, throughout the role play, gives encouragement and advice to the youth who wants to use the condom. The facilitator leads a discussion at the end of each role play about what worked and what did not work in the role play and why, including any other advice the group could give the person who wanted to use the condom.

Another activity is to develop a "Ladder of Risk." In this activity, cards are passed out to the group with individual sexual behaviors listed on them (including safe, safer, and unsafe behaviors). We also include injection drug use behaviors, such as sharing a dirty syringe, bleaching a syringe, and not sharing a syringe. The facilitator draws a ladder on a chalk board or chart pad, with "100% Risk" at the top and "100% No Risk" at the bottom. One at a time, participants are asked to tape his or her cards to the ladder where they think the activity falls in terms of the risk of HIV transmission. When all the cards are taped to the ladder, the facilitator asks the group if anyone thinks a card should be in a different spot on the ladder. The facilitator then makes adjustments to the list, as needed, and discusses each behavior and what the risks are. The facilitator leads a final discussion around how a person could minimize HIV risk by choosing a less-risky behavior.

Field Trips   In addition to the field trips mentioned earlier, we conduct HIV-specific field trips. We are fortunate in San Francisco to have several community-based agencies working on HIV issues. Our field trips have included visits to the Names Project, the organization which sponsors the AIDS quilt displays across the United States; Condomania, a condom specialty store; a theater screening of *And the Band Played On,* the HBO movie based on Randy Shilts's book; and a screening of a documentary film about women and HIV. These trips provide opportunities to engage clients in extended discussions of issues related to HIV.

Wedge Program   Wedge is a unique HIV prevention program targeting San Francisco youth. A community-initiated program started in 1986, Wedge is sponsored by the San Francisco Department of Public Health and is one of the first organized programs to present persons with AIDS as speakers in schools. When done in schools, the Wedge Program is four one-hour sessions; but given the transient nature of the LSYC population, the program is condensed to one 1.5-hour session. A Wedge educator performs a thirty-minute introductory session covering basic facts about HIV, risk behaviors for transmission, and prevention methods, including condom demonstrations. After the introduction, two HIV positive speakers, usually mixed gender, ethnicity, and sexuality, share their personal stories of how they came to be infected with HIV and what it is like living with the virus and/or disease. Depending on the language makeup of the audience, Wedge presentations are conducted in English, Spanish, or both.

The Wedge Program, and others like it, are unique in that the speakers provide a human face to the AIDS epidemic. This approach leaves no room for denial of this epidemic, and youth often spend time after the presentation making connections with the educator and the speakers about their own feelings and concerns around HIV. Studies have shown that this program has a positive effect on attitudes of adolescents towards HIV and PWAs, and youths' intention to practice HIV prevention.

Art and HIV   LSYC has been fortunate to have an artist in residence for several years, who has worked diligently to get young people to express themselves through various mediums of visual art. Often youth have expressed their feelings toward HIV in their art—commentary can be seen on the Drop-In Center ceiling tiles painted by clients, and on canvas, paper, and tile mosaics. The artist in residence also provides journal-making projects, which is another avenue for the young people to express their feelings.

As part of HIV groups, staff have used art to promote HIV prevention. We have made condom and lube earrings with beads, glitter, glue, and earring hooks; created posters with new slogans related to HIV prevention; and made collages dealing with HIV, self-esteem, and identity.

"Condom Sense" and Other Games   Games can be a great way to engage LSYC clients in HIV education and prevention techniques, such as condom use and negotiation skills. The most popular game we have for doing this education is "Condom Sense," an interactive board game designed by a former Larkin staff person. The design of the board is similar to that of Monopoly™, but is specific to Larkin Street Youth Center with names of places and actions particular to Larkin youth.

As in Monopoly™, players move their pieces around the board by rolling the die and taking actions or drawing Chance cards as instructed by the board. Youth play individually or in teams of two. Each team is given ten condoms at the beginning of the game. The purpose is to "use" all of their condoms before any other team "uses" all their own. Players use condoms by doing condom demonstrations, answering questions about HIV risk and transmission, and convincing their peers to use condoms through role plays.

Other games include "Family Feud," HIV Bingo, and Password—all variations on commonly known games. These games, however, are limited to basic HIV education. To play Family Feud, we divide clients into two or more groups and give them HIV-related questions. Points for correct questions are marked on a chalkboard, and the team with the most points at the end of a list of fifteen questions wins. The facilitator allows teams who are "behind" to catch up and to take turns answering the questions, as the purpose is not winning, but rather empowering young people to learn about and share information on HIV. HIV Bingo and Password are similar games.

Videos   Videos can be a powerful medium to provoke thought and open up discussions on HIV-related issues. Because the population is not a captive audience, the videos need to be very engaging and short and to the point. It is also helpful if the target population sees themselves reflected in the video—youth, street youth, and a multicultural youth population. Some of the videos that have worked best at Larkin include "AIDS Not Us," a fictional story involving five urban youth (primarily young African-American and Latino men); "Reality Check," a video of a multicultural population of youth providing information about the testing process and pros and cons of testing, with perspectives from both HIV positive and HIV negative youth; "Not Me: Innocence in the Time of AIDS," in which several HIV positive youth engage in a dialogue with other young people about HIV prevention and what it is like to be HIV positive. For a Spanish-speaking population, two of the favorites include "*Mi Hermano*" and "*Ojos que No Ven*," fictional stories about families and communities dealing with HIV.

One-on-One Interventions   One-on-one counseling interventions in the Drop-In Center are an important component of the HIV prevention program. Through them, we can provide specific attention and counseling targeting a particular youth's situation. Further, one-on-one interventions are an important means to reach youth who may not attend groups. This section outlines two sample interventions around HIV risk behaviors.

A female injection drug user revealed to staff that she was sharing needles with several people without cleaning them, including friends who were HIV positive. When discussing her risk for HIV transmission, she reported to staff that she "did not care." One-on-one interventions included discussing issues related to passive suicidality and a written contract between staff and the youth much like the contracts counselors make with suicidal clients. The client contracted with staff to not share needles for the following two days and to acquire a syringe for her own use. The contract also included having the youth check in with staff at least once each of these two days. This contract allowed for continued discussion around needle use and passive suicidal behaviors, as well as allowing the client to make a small but visible concrete step in behavior change.

In another instance, a gay youth reported to staff that he had begun to have sexual experiences with other men but had never used condoms, as he was uncomfortable with them and did not like the way they felt. Staff employed several one-on-one interventions with the client, showing how to eroticize latex and going over negotiation skills. Staff also screened a gay men's erotic safer-sex video for the youth and another gay male client. By the end of the interventions, the client was showing other youth how to put condoms on with their mouths, make cock rings out of the base of condoms, and advocating the use of water-based lubricants. The young man subsequently reported the practice of safer behaviors in his personal life and that two friends followed his lead.

Interventions around Injection Drug Use   Given the role of injection drug use in HIV transmission, LSYC staff employ a variety of strategies to decrease risk behaviors among the IDU population. To exchange in a dialogue with youth around their injection drug use, staff must first gain their trust—trust that we will not turn them over to authorities for illegal drug use, trust that we will not moralize on or judge their behaviors, and trust that they can turn to staff for support around HIV and drug-addiction issues related to their needle use. When a youth first arrives at the Center, he or she sees signs posted for Youth Needle Exchange, the Larkin policy for cleaning needles, and detox services. Each new client fills out an intake form, which includes several questions relating to safe needle use. Through the intake, clients are informed by staff where they can find bleach, needle exchange information, and condoms. This environment has allowed staff to more easily engage in discussions with IDU clients around safe needle usage, HIV risk behaviors, and drug addiction.

An important step in decreasing HIV transmission in this target population is to promote a culture that supports not sharing needles. In all departments of the agency, we have posted the Larkin policy on cleaning needles; this includes a bold statement that "sharing needles is *not* safe," but if youth do share needles, they should follow the cleaning instructions posted, a simplified version of the most recent guidelines from the Centers for Disease Control. Larkin has also recently collaborated with another agency in San Francisco to provide a Youth Needle Exchange once a week for the IDU street youth population. This informal needle exchange has had remarkable success in its first month, attracting some young people who have never used a needle exchange and others who only sporadically used the other needle exchange sites in the city. To attract youth to the Youth Needle Exchange, we have signs posted in all departments of the agency, reminding clients on the day that the exchange will occur, and do street outreach during the hour that the exchange is happening to further remind them to go to the site. The Youth Needle Exchange volunteer has extensive experience working with young people and has created a safe environment for them to exchange their needles. At the exchange, she distributes bleach, *Shooting Safer* manuals, and information on LSYC services and detox programs.

Shooting Safer is a manual developed by Larkin and designed for young IDUs. Written in simple language with diagrams and drawings, *Shooting Safer* provides information on how to use needles correctly to prevent health complications, how to prevent transmission of HIV and hepatitis, what to do if someone overdoses, and information on addiction and detox programs.

CONCLUSION

Effective HIV prevention education programs targeting homeless and runaway youth must address the barriers to HIV prevention behavior specific to this population. Educators need to be sensitive to the issues of these youth caught in a high-risk environment and also to the issues they have brought with them to the street. The most effective way of reducing HIV risk behavior of homeless youth is to, as LSYC's mission statement addresses, empower them to move beyond the high-risk environment of the street and to help them develop the decision-making skills, communication skills, and self-esteem necessary to reduce HIV risk in any environment.

It is also crucial that HIV prevention be provided in a continuum of services. At Larkin, helping youth exit street life and providing HIV prevention education and counseling is a team effort. From providing therapy in Case Management to providing healthy alternatives to the streets through the residential and business services, staff in all LSYC departments collaborate together to prevent the spread of HIV in the homeless youth population in San Francisco. Teamwork, perseverance, and an understanding of issues facing homeless young people provide the foundation to help youth move beyond the streets and stay safe from HIV infection.

REFERENCE

Bermudez, Ricardo, and Janet Shalwitz. (1993). "Report on HIV Seroprevalence and Transmission Factors in Young People Utilizing Special Programs for Youth Clinics." *Special Programs for Youth: A Guide to Comprehensive HIV/AIDS Services for Adolescents and Young Adults.* San Francisco: Department of Public Health, City and County of San Francisco.

9

AIDS Education: Innovative Methods for Adolescents in New Orleans

Lillian Lioeanjie

New Orleans is often described as a "gumbo," made up of many different ingredients; all sharing a common pot, yet each ingredient maintaining its own distinctive taste. Our community consists of many ethnic groups, among the oldest and most populous being African Americans. Brought to Louisiana by the French and mostly of Senegalese heritage, 500 slaves arrived in the Colony of New Orleans in 1719. Even today, after the arrival of other ethnic groups, African culture permeates all others; African Americans make up over 60 percent of New Orleans's population.

New Orleans is the second largest southern city, with a population of about 500,000. The climate is subtropical, having short winters and long, hot, and humid summers. Despite its rich cultural life, New Orleans is not an affluent city. Most residents with families earn less than $15,000 per year, making its average family income one of the lowest in the nation. Since the decline of the oil industry in the 1980s, most individuals rely on service-industry jobs in hospitals, restaurants, and hotels—often catering to tourists. The health of the New Orleans economy depends largely on whether hotels and restaurants overflow with visitors.

The only city in the nation that can boast of being a party town, New Orleans annually entertains the over one million revelers who come for Mardi Gras and other year-round festivities. It is one of the few cities where people are allowed openly to consume alcohol on the streets, especially in the French Quarter. As a result, alcoholism is a serious problem for many of its residents.

Similar to other large urban centers, New Orleans has a decaying infrastructure. As people become increasingly frustrated with poor living conditions, seeing no way out, the use of drugs (as well as the sale of drugs) provides an alternative lifestyle. Low wages, few economic opportunities, and the prevalence of drugs and their usage make New Orleans a breeding ground for high-risk behavior. Over 38,000 abandoned houses also create an ideal environment for crack users, who constitute one of the largest segments of the substance-abusing population in the city.

Because many families live in overcrowded conditions, young children are exposed to the use of drugs and alcohol. Public-housing projects contain over 15,000 residents, consisting mostly of single women who were teenage mothers or raised by teen parents. Forced to live in fear and despair with few recreational outlets for themselves or their children, too many become dependent on crack cocaine and alcohol. Their children are, therefore, frequently left to roam the streets without supervision, easy prey for sex offenders or other unscrupulous persons, making them at high risk for substance abuse and HIV infection.

The state of Louisiana has one of the poorest records pertaining to public education. Almost half of the students who enter the New Orleans public school system either drop out or fail to graduate, and illiteracy rates are high. The state ranks first in the nation for teenage drop-outs, many of whom are then unable to enter the workforce. State and local leadership have failed to give priority to its youth.

Considering the high rate of poverty in New Orleans, as well as the low literacy rate, it is no wonder that the state rates of both gonorrhea and syphilis exceed those found in the rest of the United States, and New Orleans has the highest rates of any city in Louisiana. For example, in 1993, syphilis rates in the United States as a whole were about fourteen per 100,000 population, compared to Louisiana's rate of approximately sixty-one per 100,000. Because HIV is also a sexually transmitted disease, the rapidly rising rates of gonorrhea and syphilis suggest alarming trends for the spread of HIV. Figures 9.1 and 9.2 depict the high gonorrhea and syphilis rates in Louisiana compared to the United States as a whole. Tables 9.1 and 9.2 provide an eight-year breakdown of Louisiana's gonorrhea and syphilis rates, by ethnicity.

Figure 9.1
Gonorrhea Rates, United States versus Louisiana, 1970–1993

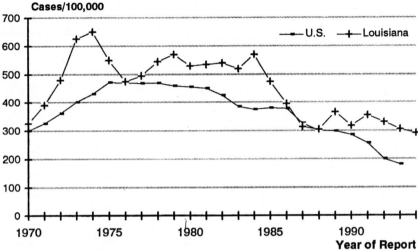

Source: Louisiana Office of Public Health.
Note: 1994 U.S. data are not available.

Table 9.1
Eight-Year Comparison of Louisiana Gonorrhea Rates, by Ethnicity

Year	White	African American	Other	Total
1987	1,525	11,645	33	13,203
1988	990	11,813	37	12,840
1989	837	14,535	34	15,406
1990	616	12,710	35	13,361
1991	864	14,021	44	14,929
1992	892	13,017	24	13,933
1993	738	12,101	54	12,893
1994	736	11,139	35	11,910

Source: STD Control, State of Louisiana. Department of Biostatistics. New Orleans, La., 1994.

National statistics indicate high infection rates for young persons in every category of STD. Adolescent girls now have the highest rates of gonorrhea in the country, and adolescent boys rank second. The rate for teenage girls is about twenty times higher than for females over thirty years of age. Approximately 10 percent of sexually active adolescent girls have been infected with gonorrhea.

Figure 9.2
P&S Syphilis Rates, United States versus Louisiana, 1970–1993

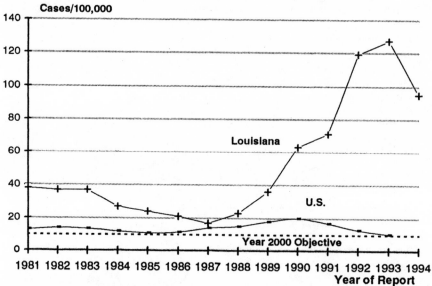

Source: Louisiana Office of Public Health.
Note: 1994 U.S. data are not available.

Table 9.2
Eight-Year Comparison of Louisiana Syphilis Rates, by Ethnicity

Year	White	African American	Other	Total
1987	82	682	2	766
1988	43	914	2	959
1989	61	1,532	5	1,598
1990	125	2,556	5	2,686
1991	130	2,872	7	3,009
1992	318	4,666	14	4,998
1993	297	5,028	16	5,341
1994	218	3,766	8	3,992

Source: STD Control, State of Louisiana. Department of Biostatistics. New Orleans, La., 1994.

This is significant, because STD infections boost the risk of contracting HIV. Many STDs have an interactive effect with HIV to enhance the transmission of both. Having an STD, such as gonorrhea, increases by as much as 100 times the chance of contracting HIV from an infected partner.

AIDS AND AFRICAN AMERICANS

The statistics for African Americans infected with HIV/AIDS are staggering. Although African Americans constitute only 12 percent of the U.S. population, 54 percent of all children with AIDS are African American, 53 percent of all women with AIDS are African American, and 32 percent of all men with AIDS are African American. Among teenagers with AIDS, more than one-third are African American. As indicated in Table 9.3, similar trends are found in the state of Louisiana.

AIDS AND YOUNG ADULTS

AIDS is also a disease of the young. According to the National Center for Health Statistics, AIDS is the sixth leading cause of death among fifteen to twenty-four year olds. More than 10,000 young adults have contracted AIDS since the start of the epidemic in the early 1980s; and, since the average incubation period for the onset of HIV is ten years, it is likely that a significant portion of young adults with AIDS contracted the disease in their teens. Of the more than 242,000 cumulative AIDS cases in the United States, 6 percent contracted the disease through heterosexual contact. However, heterosexual transmission is growing. While the medical community agrees that, besides abstinence, condom use is the most effective protection against HIV, the message is not getting through to teens. According to a study of minority youth in Detroit, only 13 percent

Table 9.3
Comparison of New Orleans Metro versus Louisiana State Cumulative AIDS Cases, by Ethnicity (as of 6/30/95)

Ethnicity	Louisiana		New Orleans Metro Area	
	Number	Percentage	Number	Percentage
White	3,873	55	2,320	56
African American	3,012	43	1,677	40
Hispanic	166	2	131	3
Asian/PI	16	0	13	0
American Indian	2	0	1	0
Unknown	10	0	7	0

Source: Louisiana Department of Public Health. HIV/AIDS Services. New Orleans, La., 1994.

Table 9.4
Comparison of New Orleans Metro versus Louisiana State Cumulative AIDS Cases, by Age

Age	Louisiana		New Orleans Metro Area	
	Number	Percentage	Number	Percentage
Under 5	55	1	45	1
5–12	12	0	6	0
13–19	61	1	25	1
20–29	1,585	22	872	21
30–39	3,206	45	1,919	46
40–49	1,477	21	901	22
Over 49	457	9	381	9

Source: Louisiana Department of Public Health. HIV/AIDS Services. New Orleans, La., 1994.

of Hispanic and 47 percent of African-American teens know that nonlatex condoms do not provide effective HIV protection. Data in Table 9.4 depict both the statewide and New Orleans Metro Area adolescent AIDS cases, by age.

As of mid-1994, adolescent HIV cases accounted for a relatively small percentage of both the state's (Louisiana) and the city's (New Orleans) AIDS cases. As of June 30, 1994, there were forty-six AIDS cases among youth thirteen to nineteen years of age in Louisiana, representing only 1 percent of the New Orleans metropolitan area total AIDS cases. However, given its long incubation period, of more relevance is the fact that 21 percent of all of the city's AIDS cases are found among those twenty to twenty-nine years old, suggesting a number of these individuals were infected while still teenagers.

All of the preceding data highlight the importance of providing AIDS education to the city's adolescent population, particularly African-American teenagers. However, developing effective strategies to work with this population poses significant challenges to health educators.

BARRIERS TO WORKING WITH ADOLESCENTS

Our experience working with teenagers, particularly "at risk" teens, has taught us that knowledge about HIV/AIDS does not necessarily translate into behavior change—either for adolescents or adults. This is especially true when substance abuse is involved.

As educators and adult role models, we sometimes believe that all teenagers are the same. This is indeed true for many aspects of adolescent behavior. Most adolescents consider themselves omnipotent, for example. Many have the attitude, "it can't happen to me," despite everything around them saying that it can. Yet we must not forget that everyone is an individual with different needs. What might be a concern for one person is not necessarily an issue for another, despite their gender and age similarities.

Providing HIV risk reduction to adolescents is also a socially sensitive endeavor. Parents and educators are concerned that, if adolescents are taught skills that require explicit sexual knowledge such as condom usage, youths will misconstrue it as a license for sexual promiscuity. Unfortunately, most school-site HIV/AIDS prevention interventions discourage condom distribution or even discussions about condom usage. Abstinence advocates believe that no sex is the only absolute way to protect adolescents.

However, it is no secret that sexual activity among adolescents in the United States is high and that early onset of sexual activity is rarely followed by a return to abstinence. The high rates of STDs and teenage pregnancy clearly indicate that a significant percentage of adolescents are having unprotected sex despite knowledge of sexually transmitted diseases, including HIV, and pregnancy. From 1981 through 1991, 24 to 30 percent of the reported morbidity from gonorrhea and 10 to 12 percent of the morbidity from primary and secondary syphilis in the United States affected adolescents.

According to the 1990 Youth at Risk Behavior Surveillance System Report by the Centers for Disease Control, African-American teens appear to be more sexually active than either their white or Hispanic counterparts. Data suggest that close to 90 percent of African-American male students, and 60 percent of African-American female high school students are sexually active. Of these, close to two-thirds (60%) of African-American males, and 20 percent of females reported having four or more sexual partners in their lifetime. Data also indicate that 50 percent of white high school students, 46 percent of Hispanic students, and 54.5 percent of African-American high school students report not using condoms during their last sexual intercourse. This trend is borne out in the rising rates of sexually transmitted diseases among adolescents. If it is true that adolescents are becoming more promiscuous, are less likely to use condoms, and are less likely to see a doctor for treatment, there is an entire class of Americans at high risk for dire health problems in the future.

Some adolescents who are HIV positive prefer to remain in school to continue to have a sense of normalcy in their lives. Often, they keep their HIV status a secret from family and close friends, believing that if it became known they would be ostracized. Some refuse to notify their sexual partners, and some admit using the virus as a form of vengeance against people. Because mandatory testing can be an infringement of rights, AIDS prevention is the best public-health policy.

However, public education efforts, particularly targeting teenagers, face significant barriers. Many teenagers believe HIV to be only a "gay disease." Many also have limited comprehension of the disease's incubation period, often view themselves as "immortal," and many are products of dysfunctional homes that are unable to provide the kind of support and advice necessary to help them make good choices. Furthermore, young girls are often victims of an ethos that says planning sex (and having protection) is the province of "bad girls." In their eyes, "good girls" get pregnant by accident—never having planned to have sex. Bad girls, by contrast, are seen as those who planned for sex and have protection. This notion is often reinforced by adults who refuse to accept that many teenagers are sexually active.

The attitudes held by teenagers about HIV/AIDS often reflect community norms and attitudes. HIV/AIDS is still seen as a gay disease in the African-American community in New Orleans. Because homosexuality is taboo, and their own perceptions of HIV as a gay disease, many African-American adults (and teens) refuse to acknowledge their risk of HIV infection. Despite outreach and education interventions, many individuals in the community, including teenagers, prefer to pretend they are not at risk. At times, it seems that the community would rather be in denial about the AIDS epidemic than acknowledge the fact that many of its members are engaging in high-risk behaviors. Furthermore, the community tends not to acknowledge its own role and responsibility in stemming the city's rate of HIV infection.

Other barriers identified by health workers are adolescent misconceptions about sexuality. These misconceptions could stem from either their environment or from the music and videos in which there are explicit sex scenes along with language that tells them that love equates with sex. Due to low reading-comprehension levels, many adolescents cannot understand some concepts. Some students do not understand, for example, the "window phase"—the period in which there are not signs or symptoms of HIV infection.

Moreover, having multiple sex partners (and unprotected sex) is not considered high-risk behavior among teens, especially if they are not gay or drug users. Such misconceptions are perpetuated by adult role models, who also refuse to recognize that HIV affects heterosexuals. These attitudes frustrate the work being done by those who are at the forefront of AIDS education.

Another barrier to providing effective health education messages to adolescents is the unwillingness to provide a credible message delivered by a credible messenger. We have learned that scare tactics, an unwillingness to recognize that many teenagers are having sex, and a refusal to use down-to-earth, explicit sexual language delivered by a credible person all present significant barriers to health education and health promotion among adolescents.

NEW ORLEANS HIV/AIDS PROGRAMS

The city's initial AIDS education program did not have a noticeable impact, particularly on teens. It consisted primarily of AIDS 101, and youth did not relate well to it. Monitoring of early implementation of the program combined with the community's response led the Health Department to consider revisions of the initial program's plan. More was needed, and the PREVAIL program was born.

In 1988, to meet the challenge of prevention, the New Orleans Health Department implemented a program that specifically targeted racial and ethnic minorities. Grasping the attention of the minority community was not an easy task. Intervention and case management services were identified as needed components to a minority initiative. The PREVAIL program of AIDS prevention was created to increase the odds that African Americans in New Orleans, and particularly African-American youth, will overcome the threat presented by AIDS. The goal of PREVAIL is to reduce the incidence and prevalence of AIDS in the African-American community. This is done by increasing the knowledge of prevention practices regarding HIV infection.

We also recognized that *who* delivers the health education message is critical to reaching adolescents. In school settings especially, we found that trust is an important requirement, and we therefore recruited and trained a number of peer educators who are able to deliver HIV/AIDS education in a responsible and accurate manner and in a language understood by their peers.

Most of the adolescents receive initial contact with the program when they come through the public-health clinic to be treated for STDs. Health staff also attempt to ascertain whether they are HIV positive—if they agree to be screened for the virus. Most prenatal exams at the public hospitals also include HIV screening. It is only through the public-health clinics and hospitals that clients are encouraged to be tested for HIV. Testing for HIV is still rarely sought out voluntarily by the age groups most at risk. Most cases of HIV remain undiagnosed, creating an even larger public-health emergency for adolescents.

OUTREACH

Health educators cannot provide HIV education if there are no clients to talk to. The first component of a successful program, therefore, is outreach, and particularly street outreach. Generally speaking, outreach should be done in teams. There is strength in numbers, both physical safety and the ability to provide information to diverse groups of youths. There are several purposes to the outreach component. First is to provide AIDS education to any youth who will listen, even if it is in a less than ideal setting (e.g., in a park or on a street corner). Second is to establish a relationship with youths, hopefully to be able to communicate with them at greater length in the community. And third is to encourage or induce youths to visit a public-health clinic or youth center where they can receive more thorough AIDS education and needed health care.

The outreach team should act in both a reactive and proactive manner. That is, the team should answer all questions by youth who seek out information from the team as well as initiate contacts with youths on the street to provide health education. In addition to HIV education, the outreach team can also hand out condoms, bleach, and other survival materials to youths who need them. Community health outreach workers, or CHOWs as they are called in some areas, should be open and friendly as well as knowledgeable. They should be people who can establish a good rapport with teens.

SCHOOL SETTINGS

Even though we are always welcome to do presentations in school settings in New Orleans, we are often not allowed to graphically describe specific sexual contacts that transmit HIV. When we are allowed to use graphic language, it is usually with the consent of school personnel. Sex-educational tools, such as puzzles and quizzes that test their knowledge (as well as coloring books for pre-adolescents) provide teens with details of how HIV can enter the body. If the teachers and faculty are cooperative, we try to make frequent visits so that students become familiar with us. Having more than one session with the same students brings trust into the relationship.

We usually use a pre-test and post-test to measure knowledge before and after an educational session. We use an instrument with twenty questions called the "Minority Quotient Questionnaire." It consists of straightforward questions that are easy to understand, and it is geared to show how African Americans perceive AIDS in the community. This and other instruments not only give us an idea of how the community at large perceives HIV/AIDS, but it also reveals some of the myths and rumors that must be addressed in order to change attitudes and behavior. We can also make use of these tools to gather information for creative games to be used at health fairs and festivals.

It is critical to emphasize here how important evaluations can be in the AIDS education process. AIDS educators always need to know whether their programs are effective—that is, reaching the target population and effecting behavior change. Local evaluations, conducted in-house or by outside evaluators, are important for making such determinations. Evaluations can tell us whether our programs are working, and whether we need to modify them.

During health fairs we usually set up a VCR, playing videos that are directed at young people. With celebrities such as Magic Johnson and Arsenio Hall, the video "Time Out" is very popular. Showing a video usually initiates discussion on a more personal level between teens and health educators. During school health fairs, students are encouraged to ask questions and are given literature that is tailored to their age group and reading levels.

Slogan and poster contests are valuable, although they can be time consuming and usually require the participation of teachers or counselors. This sometimes can pose a problem, given the fact that most school systems are overwhelmed with overcrowded classrooms and discipline problems. However, such contests can be an excellent way to get students involved in solving problems—their own and their community's. In this way, teens take ownership of the problem and become more interested and invested in helping themselves or mobilizing community prevention efforts. Slogan and poster contests require that teens take responsibility for their own health as well as the health of others.

FESTIVALS

Holding a festival is a good way of getting teens to participate. Creative games that teach or encourage them to get information about HIV can ultimately be very effective. With adolescents, as with most people, the choice to have safe sex is a choice made from moment to moment. Because increased knowledge does not always translate into behavior change, we must use innovative methods to keep people on track.

A game most people are familiar with, called "Wheel of Fortune," is commonly used at our annual health fairs. Each participant is

asked to spin the wheel and wherever the arrow points the participant must read the question and answer it. If they answer correctly,
they win a small prize. If they are wrong, the educator corrects the
participant and gives them enough information to increase their
knowledge of HIV transmission routes and prevention behaviors.
Of course, the questions that you develop for this game must come
from the concerns most often heard by health educators during their
presentations. Questions can also come from the pre- and post-test
evaluation instruments, but they must be specific to your population.

Another effective game uses cards of different colors. All cards
are face down so the participant cannot read the questions. The
participant is asked to pick up the card of his or her choice, then
answer the question under the card. When the correct answer is
given, comments may be made by the facilitator or educator and the
participant is thanked for participating. If an incorrect answer is
given, anyone else playing is encouraged to answer. If no one can
answer correctly, the educator answers the question and clarifies
anything that may seem unclear to the participants. It is important
never to embarrass people who give wrong answers; it is equally
critical to praise the person who knows the correct answer. Adolescents are thus made to value information and remember what they
have learned. So as not to trivialize the process, it may be better not
to give a prize unless it is in response to HIV/AIDS awareness. An
example of an appropriate prize—one that we have used successfully—is a trophy of the world. On it would be written "Thanks for
Helping Combat HIV/AIDS in the World." Health fairs or informal
gatherings are also good places to solicit participation for panel or
group discussions. Appealing to teens for their input as volunteers to
help in the prevention of this epidemic has proven very beneficial.

We believe that it is sometimes useful to provide incentives for
participation in HIV education. We do whatever it takes to get youths
to listen. A wide variety of incentives seem to work, depending on
the level of participation of the youth (and the budget of the agency).
A simple candy bar can be sufficient for minimal involvement. For
a larger project or for longer-term involvement, a gift certificate to
the movies or an article of clothing would be appropriate. It is important to note, however, that incentives are best used to get
someone's attention. It is up to the health educator to do the rest.

Most of the interventions that have been discussed relate primarily to one-time or short-term interventions. It would be desirable
for health educators to work with youths over an extended period
of time. If possible, therefore, an HIV education program should
have a case management component. That is, the program should,

when feasible, keep detailed data on clients. The data can be used both for clinical and case management purposes. Over several interventions with a particular youth, the health educator can go into greater depth about various aspects of AIDS education. Moreover, the educator can make appropriate referrals; for example, to the Department of Public Health, a teen drop-in center, a runaway shelter, and the like. These supplemental interventions can, in turn, reinforce the AIDS education message you are trying to impart.

CONCLUSION

Educating adolescents about the dangers of HIV/AIDS poses many challenges. Included among these are the following: (1) HIV/AIDS is often seen as a gay disease among African-American adults and teens; (2) adolescents do not see themselves reflected in AIDS statistics because of a lack of understanding about the disease's incubation period. Many teenagers see themselves as immortal and not at risk for anything, including HIV/AIDS; (3) there is a general distrust of government by the African-American community; (4) many schools will not allow frank, open discussions of sex and its relationship to HIV; and, (5) the African-American community has not yet adopted a proactive role to stopping the spread of HIV in the community.

Yet, our work in New Orleans has shown us that adolescents can be reached effectively by keeping the following issues in mind. First, it is important to remember that one method alone, or even two or three, may not achieve the desired results. Adolescents, like many other populations, are not monolithic, and different approaches may be effective with different groups of adolescents. We have tried a variety of strategies, including health fairs, poster contests, festivals, games, videos, peer educators, group discussions, and prevention case management.

Second, adolescents most at risk of HIV infection are often difficult to reach. They are often homeless, have dropped out of school, have low self-esteem, and may be exchanging sex for money or drugs in order to survive. Special approaches such as prevention case management may be the most effective way to work with these youths.

Third, the message and messenger are both critical to success of any health education approach. The strategies used must be culturally relevant and appropriate for the audience. For example, we found that peer educators were able to most effectively communicate with their peers. Three integral and equally important components of effective prevention programs are framing the prevention message, developing effective communication strategies, and accessing the target population.

And fourth, while we know that imparting knowledge alone rarely changes behavior, in order to create an intervention that is able to help individuals change their high-risk behaviors, they must first receive accurate information from a source they trust. For African Americans, moreover, ethnically based values of cooperation and unity may be more powerful motivators of behavior change than strict appeals to individualistic action. HIV prevention programs in the African-American community require long-term interventions that focus on ensuring the long-term health of the community.

10

Contextualizing the Development of Adolescent Girls: The Missing Piece in HIV Education

Mary Bentley and
Kathryn Herr

This chapter is devoted to prevention of HIV-related behaviors in girls. Current epidemiological data show trends that have signaled a need to focus on the unique needs of adolescent girls. We make the case here that literature emerging from the fields of adolescent development and feminist theory have not yet been connected with the education of girls around decreasing risk of HIV infection. Taking into account the unique psychosocial needs of girls during this period of development when they are at highest risk would enhance the effectiveness of programs and perhaps reduce the incidence of HIV infection in women and children. The history of this tragic epidemic has been laced with political silencing and questionable medical ethics. We are at a critical juncture where we can no longer keep girls silent; in fact, this may be jeopardizing their very survival.

TRENDS IN ADOLESCENT HIV INFECTION

An important factor related to early adolescent teens is that over 20 percent of all individuals with AIDS are in their twenties (CDC, 1990a). The average length of time between HIV infection and the development of full-blown AIDS is approximately ten years; it must therefore be assumed that the majority of these people became infected during adolescence. Data indicate that, between 1989 and 1990, teenage AIDS cases increased 51 percent. It is projected that the number of teenage AIDS cases will double annually (Stanton et al., 1990; Burkhart, 1991). With the aforementioned latency period of ten years, this trend also indicates an increase in HIV transmission within the pre-teen and early teen populations (Stine, 1993).

The following are the cumulative totals of AIDS cases between October 1991 and September 1993 for males and females aged thirteen to nineteen, based on their exposure group. These cases represent less than 1 percent of all diagnosed AIDS cases for males, and approximately 1 percent of all diagnosed cases for females. While these may seem like relatively small numbers, they do not accurately portray adolescent risk, due to the ten-year latency period (DiClemente, 1992). Nationally, AIDS was the tenth leading cause of death between 1984 and 1987 for individuals aged fifteen to twenty-four. By 1987, AIDS became the sixth leading cause of death for this age group (Kilbourne et al., 1990). Between July 1988 and July 1989, the CDC noted a 43 percent increase in the number of identified AIDS cases among adolescents (CDC, 1991).

Teens who are members of an ethnic minority are disproportionately affected by AIDS. The most heavily affected groups of teens are African American and Hispanic American. African Americans represent 26 percent of all adult AIDS cases and 58 percent of all pediatric AIDS cases (Heyward and Curran, 1988; Morgan and Curran, 1986), and Hispanic Americans represent 14 percent of all adult AIDS cases and 22 percent of all pediatric cases (Schinke et al., 1990). DiClemente (1992:328) states, "Multicultural populations, especially Blacks and Latinos, are disproportionately represented among AIDS cases, even among adolescents ages 13–19."

In addition, there seems to be a clear difference in the ways in which boys and girls are becoming infected. Table 10.1 indicates that transmission via heterosexual contact accounted for 3 to 4 percent of the AIDS cases in males between 1991 and 1993, while it accounted for 50 to 54 percent of all cases in females during this same time period. Most girls are becoming infected by having sex with boys who are infected, and boys are becoming infected from having sex with other boys who are infected. Heterosexual trans-

Table 10.1
AIDS Cases in Adolescents and Adults under Age Twenty-Five, by Sex and Exposure Category (Reported October 1991 through September 1992, October 1992 through September 1993, and Cumulative Totals through 1993, United States)

Age Group 13–19, Cumulative Totals (10/91–9/93)	Number	Percentage	
Male Exposure Groups			
Men who have sex with men	319	33.0	
Injecting drug use	62	6.0	
Men who have sex with men and inject drugs	45	5.0	
Hemophilia or coagulation disorder	440	45.0	
Heterosexual contact	29	3.0	
Receipt of blood transfusion, blood components, or tissue	42	4.0	
Risk not identified	40	4.0	
Female Exposure Groups			
Injecting drug use	86	20.0	
Hemophilia or coagulation disorder	5	1.0	
Heterosexual contact	236	54.0	
Sex with infected drug user		127	53.8
Sex with HIV-infected person		76	32.2
Receipt of blood transfusion, blood components, or tissue	41	9.0	
Risk not identified	67	15.0	
Age Group 20–24, Cumulative Totals (10/91–9/93)			
Male Exposure Groups			
Men who have sex with men	6,485	64.0	
Injecting drug use	1,245	12.0	
Men who have sex with men and inject drugs	1,063	11.0	
Hemophilia or coagulation disorder	385	4.0	
Heterosexual contact	363	4.0	
Receipt of blood transfusion, blood components, or tissue	85	1.0	
Risk not identified	445	4.0	
Female Exposure Groups			
Injecting drug use	931	35.0	
Hemophilia or coagulation disorder	9	0.0	
Heterosexual contact	1,329	50.0	
Sex with infected drug user		754	56.7
Sex with HIV-infected person		357	26.9
Receipt of blood transfusion, blood components, or tissue	81	3.0	
Risk not identified	291	11.0	

Source: CDC, 1993, p. 10, graph titled "AIDS cases in adolescents and adults under age 25, by sex and exposure category, reported October 1991 through September 1993, and cumulative totals through 1993, United States."

mission in girls is also accompanied by issues of teen pregnancy, other STD transmission, and is tragically linked to the increase in pediatric AIDS. It seems clear that prevention and programmatic efforts need to focus on the very unique and pressing needs of adolescent girls.

The current call for HIV education for young people comes at a time when there is a growing body of knowledge about the unique developmental pathways of adolescent girls. As there is a move from monolithic conceptualizations of "normal" development, early adolescence is increasingly seen as a time of heightened vulnerability for girls, comparable to the period of early childhood for boys. "Yet despite the repeated reports of what would seem to be a startling asymmetry between the vulnerability of girls and boys to environmental stress or insult, this difference in boys' and girls' development remains essentially unexplained and unexplored theoretically" (Mikel Brown and Gilligan, 1990:5–6). Since girls are of school age during this period of crisis in development, it becomes an educational as well as a psychological issue: How do we allow this new information about developmental differences to inform our thinking about education, in this case HIV education, and appropriate interventions?

FEMALE EARLY ADOLESCENT DEVELOPMENT

Seen as one of the cornerstones in the developmental literature, the work of Erik Erikson (1968) has informed much of what we consider we know about the developmental life cycle and the state of adolescence in particular. More recent work has begun to recast this stage of development and bring different lenses to developmental schema. For example, Newman and Newman (1987) differentiate between the tasks of early and later adolescence, treating these periods as unique in their own right, rather than one long continuum of identity development. Recent thought in education (Carnegie Council on Adolescent Development, 1989), under the rubric of middle-level education, is making the ages nine through fourteen distinct, separating them from the frames of both elementary and secondary schooling.

In terms of female adolescent development, the work of Carol Gilligan, among others, has been pivotal in beginning to document the developmental pathways of girls. While there is evidence of what has been traditionally conceived of as a move toward being more autonomous, differentiated from others, and less dependent on authority, there are indications simultaneously of a loss of voice, a struggle to speak with authority, and a replacement of real relationships with an idealized version of relating that renders a girl mute in regard to expressing her authentic thoughts and feelings. While much of Gilligan's research (Mikel Brown and Gilligan, 1990; Gilligan et al., 1990) has focused primarily on middle- to upper-class Caucasian girls, others are beginning to extend her initial research into a broader population (see, for example, Robinson and Ward, 1991; Kim, 1991).

In their longitudinal work, Mikel Brown and Gilligan (1990) find that girls ages seven through ten speak openly about their thoughts and feelings; they remain "authentic" to themselves, working to be heard even if it means sailing into conflict in terms of their relationships. Younger girls feel entitled to be heard and live their relational lives accordingly. Intruding around early adolescence is the specter of the "perfect girl": "the girl who has no bad thoughts or feelings, the kind of person everyone wants to be with; worthy of praise and attention, worthy of inclusion and love . . . the girl who speaks quietly, calmly, who is always nice and kind, never mean or bossy" (Mikel Brown and Gilligan, 1990:16).

Separating herself from what she knows and feels, the early adolescent girl works to transform herself into the girl she thinks others want her to be. To be herself and to speak her mind and heart with authority is seen as too risky, making her too vulnerable in her "imperfection" to the rejection of others. "Girls at the edge of adolescence struggle with images of perfection and idealized relationships in which to care for themselves is often characterized by them as 'bad,' 'selfish,' or 'wrong'." The girls become "unsure of the accuracy of their perceptions, afraid that speaking up will damage relationships or compromise their image in the eyes of others" (Mikel Brown and Gilligan, 1990:7). Ironically, this image maintenance results in girls disconnecting from authentic relationships and working instead for ones characterized as peaceful, smooth running, and void of conflict. The price paid for these conflict-free relationships is the silencing of their voices; no longer knowing what it was they knew during their younger years (i.e., that the way to authentic connection is in speaking one's heart and mind even in the face of potential conflict). They have, in essence, removed themselves from relationships at the very time they desire and need connection.

A girl's developmental pathway to identity formation diverges from that of boys; instead of a model of separation and individuation, she instead develops a sense of herself as a "being-in relation," "developing all of one's self in increasingly complex ways, in increasingly complex relationships" (Miller, 1991:20). This self-in-relation model of female development posits that, for girls and women, "the primary experience of self is relational, that is, the self is organized and developed in the context of important relationships" (Surrey, 1991:52).

Self-esteem for females correlates to the degree of emotional shar-ing, openness, and mutual sense of understanding and regard in a relational context (Surrey, 1991). In measures of self-esteem, girls take a precipitous plunge when they enter middle school; boys seem to maintain their strong sense of self-esteem because "they feel ca-pable of 'doing things'" (Sadker and Sadker, 1994:79). A girl's sense of self-esteem and competence is often bound to experiencing emo-tional connection and feeling effective in relationships (Miller, 1991), making this decision to disconnect from authentic relationships one with devastating repercussions for early adolescent girls. The up-shot is that choosing between being "selfish" and "bad" or being silent is no choice at all, resulting in a period of developmental crisis for early adolescent girls. "If one considers self-authorization, self-knowledge, clarity, courage, openness, and free-flowing con-nections with others and the world as signs of psychological health or development, then these girls are in fact not developing, but show evidence of loss, struggle and signs of an impasse in their ability to act in the face of conflict" (Mikel Brown and Gilligan, 1990:7).

THE DEVELOPMENT OF THE FEMALE SEXUAL SELF

While there is no real body of research literature dealing with fe-male adolescent sexual desire, the process of documenting the so-cietal silence surrounding this issue has begun (Tolman, 1991; Fine, 1993). The impact of this missing discourse may result in girls' fail-ure to know themselves as the subjects of their own sexuality, and may limit their sense of agency around sexual decision making (Fine, 1993; Tolman, 1991; Miller, 1991). Espin (1984, cited in Ward and Taylor, 1992) posits that when girls speak of being "swept away" in a moment of passion it is perhaps a reflection of traditional cultural values that say girls should not know, feel, or learn about their sexu-ality. "If girls could conceive of themselves as sexual subjects, they could then potentially make decisions about their sexual behavior and experience that would be healthy for them" (Tolman, 1991:59).

In regard to sexuality, most girls still learn that their own sexual percep-tions, sensations and impulses are not supposed to arise from themselves but are to be brought forth by and for men. . . . The girl picks up the strong message that her own perceptions about her bodily and sexual feelings are not acceptable. They acquire connotations of badness and evil. They be-come parts of herself that are shameful and wrong. . . . In the face of this, the solution of "doing it for others" can seem to offer a ready answer. The problem is that this solution is one that attempts to leave her—and her sense of herself—with all of her own psychological construction—out of the relationship. (Miller, 1991:19–20)

The work of Miller highlights the needs of adolescent girls to use all of their capacities, including the sexual capacity, but to do so within the larger desire to enhance "being-in-relationship." She traces the altering of girls as active agents transformed to selves who must defer to others' needs or desires in the name of preserving "relationships." Adolescent girls often attempt to solve problems in relationships by silencing themselves, avoiding conflict and disagreement but also, in essence, withdrawing themselves from authentic connections (Mikel Brown and Gilligan, 1990).

In her work on female sexuality, Judith Jordan (1987, cited in Tolman, 1991) outlines a model of "contextual desire," where the central dynamic of female sexuality is relational: She describes this as a desire to experience a joining together in such a way where the joining becomes "greater than the separate selves." She sees this as sexuality informed by empathetic knowing of each other, experienced by the girl as being "emotionally held."

THE DIVERGENCE OF THE MALE SEXUAL SELF

The development of a male sense of self and identity is fostered through an emphasis on early emotional separation and difference. Surrey points out that this assertion of difference fosters a basic relational stance of disconnection and disidentification: "For boys then, 'separation' means not only a simple physical but an emotional disconnection, often with the goal of not being bound or 'controlled' by mother's feeling states or needs. For girls, 'being present with' psychologically is experienced as self-enhancing, whereas for boys it may come to be experienced as invasive, engulfing or threatening" (1991:55).

The developmental schema for boys emphasizes separation and individuation as the basic goal for self-exploration and growth; looking at girls through a self-in-relation lens, the deepening capacity for relationships and relational competence are keys in the growing sense of self. Miller, reflecting on this seeming collision of developmental pathways of adolescent girls and boys, contextualizes it in the following way:

She wishes that the other person would be able to enter into a relationship. . . . I believe that the boy really has the same needs, at bottom. However, he has been much more preoccupied with trying to develop himself and a sense of his independent identity. The culture has made the very heavy demand that he be so preoccupied. It has been doing so all along, but it does so at adolescence in an even more forceful way. (1991:20)

Coupled with this enhanced sense of the male self as individual is the false premise that hormones in males create a more powerful sex drive than in females; a drive that males can barely control. As Whatley (1992) points out, this misrepresentation of the biological facts, seen in conjunction with the silence around female sexual desire, forms the basis for much of the sexual double standard. Girls then become responsible for not only their own sexuality but that of males as well. Her roles include being careful not to "lead him on" and learning to say "no" to "unwanted" sexual advances; failing that, she is to take responsibility for contraception or bear the consequences.

The playing field for sexual activity is thus laid. Males, disconnected from a sense of relationships and taught to value the individual self, experience the cultural construction of their sexuality as a force virtually beyond their control. Girls, hoping for authentic connection, seek a joining that is larger than the separate selves; sex becomes a potential place for the emotional holding they desire. Girls fall silent as active agents in the construction of relationships, deferring to others' wants and needs in the hope of being able to maintain the connection. At the very time that girls have virtually lost their voices, they are held accountable in their sexual lives for using them: "just say no" or experience the consequences. Ironically, while much intervention has focused on the consequences end of the spectrum—teen pregnancy and HIV infection—little in the literature links intervention back to the developmental crisis of girls: how to help girls give voice to their own needs and desires, how to break the silence about female desire and help girls claim themselves as sexual beings, and how to reframe the construction of being "selfish" in relationships to one of being an agent on their own behalf.

THE CURRENT STATE OF SEXUALITY EDUCATION

While there is a strong national consensus in favor of HIV/AIDS education for young people, issues of the timing of such education, as well as what should be included in the curriculum, continue to be controversial. Over half of the states have mandated HIV/AIDS education for young people, but fewer than one-third of metropolitan school districts offer at least one class period of sexuality education to the majority of their student bodies before the ninth grade (Silin, 1992). While the majority of students report having taken a sexuality education course by age nineteen, a significant number of youth are sexually active before their first formal encounter with the subject matter (Marsiglio and Mott, 1986, cited in Sears, 1992). Sexuality education is most commonly offered in ninth or tenth grade, presented as a separate unit in classes such as home economics, physical education, science, or health (Sears, 1992).

A study of over 750 eighth grade students in rural school districts found that almost 70 percent of boys and 40 percent of girls had engaged in sexual intercourse (Alexander et al., 1989, cited in Sears, 1992); in a study of inner-city students, 92 percent of ninth grade boys and 54 percent of ninth grade girls were sexually active (Zabin et al., 1986, cited in Sears, 1992). Given adolescents' current rates of contracting other sexually transmitted diseases and their contraceptive histories, their behaviors put them at high risk for HIV infection (Brooks-Gunn, 1992). As Sears (1992) points out, the current placement of sexuality education in the school curriculum does not parallel students' needs and concerns.

State-approved HIV curricula usually emphasize information about healthy lifestyles, communicable diseases, HIV transmission and prevention, and reproductive biology, particularly the female aspects. Abstinence is clearly the preventive measure of choice among educators, and decision making "has become a code phrase for a 'Just say no' message" (Silin, 1992:268). Many school districts put constraints on the discussion of subjects such as contraception and safer sex that might be construed as encouraging sexual activity. In addition, "discussions of value laden topics such as criteria for determining acceptable types of sexual activities; feelings of sexual arousal, desire and pleasure; dynamics of power in sexual relationships; and reproductive control (among others) are almost totally ignored in middle and high school sexuality education classes" (Sapon-Shevin and Goodman, 1992:99).

Current curricular approaches tend to isolate sexuality and its potential outcomes from the context of human relationships; much of sexuality education is based on a traditional understanding of the central tasks of adolescence; that is, separation, individuation, and independence.

Traditional sexuality education programs reflect the privileging of individuality and independence by stressing as a marker of maturity, autonomous sexual decision making (determining and asserting one's own personal values along with taking personal responsibility for managing one's own sexuality). Not only does this view of development leave out the way adolescent girls experience the world and make decisions, but it also disregards cultural variation in sexual decision making. (Ward and Taylor, 1992:195)

More recent conceptualizations, then, of girls' development call into question the current timing and direction of sexuality education and raise a serious challenge to educators and others working for HIV prevention.

RISK TAKING AND ADOLESCENT DEVELOPMENT

HIV prevention efforts have been conceptually fixed on approaching the adolescent as a vulnerable vessel that gets filled with risks. The National Commission on AIDS (1993) echoes this as the adolescent experience. "One of the major developmental tasks necessary for teens to accomplish on their way to adulthood is emancipation and independence from their families. Pushing boundaries, testing limits, and questioning adult authority are ways for young people to move into adulthood. While risk-taking behavior is a natural part of adolescent experience, the presence of HIV makes sexual and drug-taking behaviors particularly dangerous today" (1994:6). Hence, the goal of HIV education is to reduce these risks that adolescents take on as a natural part of their development. Risk-reduction curriculums are often designed to assist students in the development of decision-making skills, enabling them to have the ability to make informed decisions about risks they can choose to incur. This again represents the decontextualization of their experience, and discounts developmental differences that may cause girls to loose voice.

Traditional theorists believe that early adolescence is marked by very concrete thinking, with an inability to project oneself into the future. "They [early adolescents] are less able to see the implications of their actions on their futures, and also are less able to take responsibility for their actions and the consequences of their actions when they occur" (Howard, 1993:84). There is, however, an alternative reality concerning adolescent risk taking that is emerging in health education literature. One researcher asked 199 adolescents and their parents to access the relative risk involved in a variety of specified activities. It was concluded that adolescents and their parents assessed the risks in very similar ways; hence the notion that all adolescents fail to assess personal risk appropriately is being questioned. Another critical voice of this developmental period of invulnerability argues, "For some young people, particularly the most disenfranchised minority youth, it is not personal invulnerability that is operative, but rather a loss of hope for the future" (Fullilove, 1991).

These emerging paradigms have presented an alternative lens through which adolescent risk taking can be viewed. Alternatives to the traditional developmental theories about adolescents shift the theoretical underpinnings of programs and curriculums designed to reduce risk. If alternative developmental theories concerning the unique pathway of adolescent girls were used as the theoretical basis of prevention programs, it would certainly transform curriculum, practice, and program planning to reflect a wider range of developmental experience. This provides a radically different base from which to confront the increasing number of HIV-infected adolescent girls. Rather than accepting the reality that this is a vulnerable population incurring dangerous risks as a part of their development, we need to consider what unique developmental needs they may be satisfying by engaging in high-risk behaviors.

RECONCEPTUALIZING HIV EDUCATION IN THE CONTEXT OF SCHOOL REFORM

It is impossible to reconceptualize sexuality and HIV prevention education that would consider the unique developmental pathways of girls without situating it in the larger context of schooling for girls. While there is a growing body of literature that documents how the current construction of schooling disenfranchises and silences girls (Sadker and Sadker, 1994; American Association of University Women, 1991), there is also a growing movement to rethink educational structures, particularly at the middle school level, informed by current developmental theory (Carnegie Council on Adolescent Development, 1989).

While there is considerable work yet to be done to integrate into mainstream developmental theory the newer work by Gilligan and others on female development, the current direction of school reform could provide just such an opportunity. Many of the middle school reform efforts, while not explicitly grounded in a gender analysis of schooling, are nonetheless directions that potentially benefit girls. For example, many middle schools are moving toward "family groupings" and faculty–student advisement systems that foster an atmosphere of supportive, nurturing relationships; now that it is known that a girl's sense of self is fostered in relationships, family groupings and advising are structurally conducive to enhancing this female developmental pathway. The task for schools, then, is not only to rethink curriculum based on current developmental theory, but to rethink fundamental school structures in ways that honor a student body that is male and female, as well as diverse in terms of culture and social class.

In terms of sexuality education, the formal curriculum is obviously only one avenue for information. As students work to make meaningful decisions regarding their own sexual identities and behaviors, they do so in a school culture that has been documented as

one that is both homophobic and a site for blatant sexual harassment (Bogart and Stein, 1987). In addition, school structures are
often hierarchical, perpetuating a power-over model of leadership
with men more typically in administrative roles (Shakeshaft, 1987).
Unless sexuality education is conceptualized as a school-wide effort, rather than a narrow, specialized curricular strand, the formal-
ized messages of the classroom will continue to be offset by the
realities of the larger social context of the school.

While initially appearing unrelated to HIV prevention, school practices designed to encourage girls' voices and nurture retention of their
authentic selves should correlate to girls' sense of agency in terms of
sexual decision making. Sadker and Sadker (1994) document how boys
systematically receive more teacher time, attention, and practice solving complex problems than their female counterparts. Simply making
the educational playing field even would be one step in fostering an
environment conducive to girls' learning and development.

The structure of relationships within the adult community of the
school also models to girls the possibilities open to them in terms
of having voice; or, conversely, being silenced. Dorney (forthcoming) asserts that it is impossible to solicit girls' voices without recti-
fying the silencing that occurs among female educators in schools;
she makes explicit the linkages between the possibilities offered
female adults and those perceived as options by girls. Women educators must come to terms with their own images of how they must
behave and be (i.e., the adult version of the "perfect girl") in order
to begin to explore more authentic roles with girls.

Voice training by adults, especially adult "good women," rein-
forces these images of female perfection—"nice girls" are always
calm, controlled, and quiet—they never cause a ruckus; they are
never noisy, bossy, or aggressive; they are not anxious and do not
cause trouble (Mikel Brown and Gilligan, 1990:19). In other words,
they are not authentic self-agents empowered to make decisions on
their own behalf.

The historical record documents that narrow approaches to the
control of sexually transmitted diseases have failed (Silin, 1992);
virtually absent from conventional sexuality education is the study
of the social and psychological contexts within which young adolescents become sexual beings (Sapon-Shevin and Goodman, 1992).
Yet sexuality education itself is "socially constructed in that it is
created within a political and social context that includes the dynamic interplay of race, gender and class oppression" (Ward and
Taylor, 1992:183). "Preventing the transmission of HIV involves not
only learning about condoms and spermicides and negotiating sex;

it also means developing tools of political analysis, a commitment to social change, and an ethic of caring and responsibility. In short, we must shift our attention from HIV prevention narrowly defined as a means of behavioral control to a broader focus that would more accurately reflect our students' life worlds" (Silin, 1992:278).

Silin goes on to suggest that effective sexuality education is education that empowers students, decreasing their sense of vulnerability as we encourage their sense of agency and entitlement; it must be based on the voices of students as they work to articulate their experiences in their social contexts. It means that we, as educators, must be willing to elicit their voices and listen when they speak.

CONCLUSION

We have attempted in this chapter to apply recent developmental theory to a population that is increasingly appearing in epidemiological data regarding HIV infection. We are suggesting that the current trends in prevention have not taken into account the unique developmental pathways of early adolescent girls. Until we design program strategies and interventions that have, at their core, the development of girls and their social cultural context, we can expect this tragic increase in infection to continue.

Perhaps before we can really begin to find solutions to the issues facing HIV prevention, we must continue to muddy the waters. When AIDS first appeared in the United States it was linked to the gay man. As the disease progressed, it proved itself to be a disease incurred through specific behaviors. As we have attempted to clear these and other myths concerning who is susceptible, we have new evidence that girls may be at a critical developmental period during the time they are becoming sexually active and incurring risk. Perhaps prevention efforts for girls would be more effective if the developmental motivations for becoming sexually active could be met in other ways. Eliciting and listening to the voices of girls could offer some insight into these motivations.

The redesigning of middle schools and the retraining of professionals to include developmental pathways that are unique to girls may be more effective at addressing the root cause of the increase in HIV among girls than the current trends of risk reduction. We cannot afford to be homophobic, racist, or sexist in our approach to this disease. The reexamination of what we assume to be true about development, and the move away from monolithic conceptualizations, could be the most critical step in creating programs that can foster healthy resistance in all children, including girls.

REFERENCES

American Association of University Women Educational Foundation. (1991). *Shortchanging Girls. Shortchanging America.* Washington, D.C.: American Association of University Women Educational Foundation.

Bogart, K., and N. Stein. (1987). Breaking the Silence: Sexual Harassment in Education. *Peabody Journal of Education* 64(4): 146–163.

Brooks-Gunn, J. (1992). The Impact of Puberty and Sexual Activity upon the Health and Education of Adolescent Girls and Boys. In *Sex Equity and Sexuality in Education*, edited by S. Klein, 97–126. New York: State University of New York Press.

Burkhart, D. (1991). Who Said the Sexual Revolution Is Over? *Medical Aspects of Human Sexuality* 25: 9.

Carnegie Council on Adolescent Development. (1989). *Turning Points: Preparing Youth for the 21st Century.* New York: Carnegie Corporation.

Centers for Disease Control (CDC). (1990). *HIV/AIDS Surveillance: August.* Atlanta: CDC.

Centers for Disease Control (CDC). (1991). *Division of STD/HIV Prevention Annual Report, 1990.* Atlanta: CDC.

Centers for Disease Control (CDC). (1993). *HIV/AIDS Surveillance Report.* Atlanta: CDC.

DiClemente, R. L. (1992). Epidemiology of AIDS, HIV Prevalence, and HIV Incidence among Adolescents. *Journal of School Health* 62(7): 325–330.

Dorney, J. (forthcoming). Educating toward Resistance: A Task for Women Teaching Girls. *Youth and Society.*

Erikson, E. (1968). *Identity, Youth and Crisis.* New York: W. W. Norton.

Fine, M. (1993). Sexuality, Schooling and Adolescent Females: The Missing Discourse of Desire. In *Beyond Silenced Voices: Class, Race and Gender in United States Schools*, edited by L. Weiss and M. Fine, 77–99. New York: State University of New York Press.

Fullilove, M. (1991). Testimony before the National Commission on AIDS: Adolescents and HIV Disease. 13 March, Chicago.

Gilligan, C., N. Lyons, and T. Hanmer. (1990). *Making Connections: The Relational Worlds of Adolescent Girls at Emma Willard School.* Cambridge: Harvard University Press.

Hessol, N. A., G. W. Rutherford, A. R. Lifson, et al. (1988). "The Natural History of HIV Infection in a Cohort of Homosexual and Bisexual Men: A Decade of Follow-Up." Proceedings of the IV International Conference on AIDS, Stockholm, Sweden, abstract 4096.

Heyward, W. L., and J. W. Curran. (1988). The Epidemiology of AIDS in the U.S. *Scientific American* 259(4): 72–81.

Howard, M. (1993). Testimony before the National Commission on AIDS: Prevention Strategies in the Workplace and Schools: Current Challenges. 11 March, Austin, Texas.

Kilbourne, B. W., J. W. Buehler, and M. F. Rogers. (1990). AIDS as a Cause of Death in Children, Adolescents, and Young Adults. *American Journal of Public Health* 80(4): 499–550.

Kim, H. (1991). Do You Have Eyelashes? In *Women, Girls and Psychotherapy: Reframing Resistance,* edited by C. Gilligan, A. Rogers, and D. Tolman, 201–212. New York: Haworth Press.

Mikel Brown, L., and C. Gilligan. (1990). The Psychology of Women and the Development of Girls. Paper presented at the annual meeting of the American Educational Research Association.

Miller, J. (1991). The Development of Women's Sense of Self. In *Women's Growth in Connection: Writings from the Stone Center,* edited by J. Jordan, A. Kaplan, J. Miller, I. Stiver, and J. Surrey, 11–26. New York: Guilford Press.

Morgan, W. M., and J. W. Curran. (1986). Acquired Immunodeficiency Syndrome: Current and Future Trends. *Public Health Reports* 101: 459–465.

National Commission on AIDS. (1993). *Preventing HIV/AIDS in Adolescents.* Washington, D.C.: National Commission on AIDS.

Newman, B., and P. Newman. (1987). *Development through Life: A Psychosocial Approach.* Chicago: Dorsey Press.

Robinson, T., and J. Ward. (1991). A Belief in Self Far Greater than Anyone's Disbelief: Cultivating Resistance among African American Female Adolescents. In *Women, Girls and Psychotherapy: Reframing Resistance,* edited by C. Gilligan, A. Rogers, and D. Tolman. New York: Haworth Press.

Sadker, M., and D. Sadker. (1994). *Failing at Fairness: How America's Schools Cheat Girls.* New York: Charles Scribner's Sons.

Sapon-Shevin, M., and J. Goodman. (1992). Learning to Be the Opposite Sex: Sexuality Education and Sexual Scripting in Early Adolescence. In *Sexuality and the Curriculum: The Politics and Practices of Sexuality Education,* edited by J. Sears, 89–105. New York: Teachers' College Press.

Schinke, S. P., G. J. Botvin, M. A. Orlandi, R. P. Schilling, and A. N. Gordon. (1990). African-American and Hispanic-American Adolescents, HIV Infection, and Preventive Intervention. *AIDS Education and Prevention* 2(4): 305–312.

Sears, J. (1992). Dilemmas and Possibilities of Sexuality Education: Reproducing the Body Politic. In *Sexuality and the Curriculum: The Politics and Practices of Sexuality Education,* edited by J. Sears, 7–33. New York: Teachers' College Press.

Shakeshaft, C. (1987). *Women in Educational Administration.* Beverly Hills, Calif.: Sage.

Silin, J. (1992). School Based HIV/AIDS Education: Is There Safety in Safer Sex? In *Sexuality and the Curriculum: The Politics and Practices of Sexuality Education,* edited by J. Sears, 267–283. New York: Teachers' College Press.

Stanton, B., M. Black, V. Keane, and S. Feigelman. (1990). HIV Risk Behaviors in Young Black People: Can We Benefit from 30 Years of Research Experience? *AIDS and Public Policy Journal* 5: 17–23.

Stine, G. (1993). *Acquired Immune Deficiency Syndrome: Biological, Medical, Social, and Legal Issues.* Englewood Cliffs, N.J.: Prentice-Hall.

Surrey, J. (1991). The Self-in-Relation: A Theory of Women's Development. In *Women's Growth in Connection: Writings from the Stone Center*, edited by J. Jordan, A. Kaplan, J. Miller, I. Stiver, and J. Surrey, 51–66. New York: Guilford Press.

Tolman, D. (1991). Adolescent Girls, Women and Sexuality: Discerning Dilemmas of Desire. In *Women, Girls, and Psychotherapy: Reframing Resistance*, edited by C. Gilligan, A. Rogers, and D. Tolman, 55–69. New York: Haworth Press.

Ward, J., and J. Taylor. (1992). Sexuality Education for Immigrant and Minority Students: Developing a Culturally Appropriate Curriculum. In *Sexuality and the Curriculum: The Politics and Practices of Sexuality Education*, edited by J. Sears, 183–202. New York: Teachers' College Press.

Whatley, M. (1992). Goals for Sex-Equitable Sexuality Education. In *Sex Equity and Sexuality in Education*, edited by S. Klein, 83–95. New York: State University of New York Press.

11

HIV Education and the Sexual Assault Survivor

Elizabeth R. Cocina and
Cassandra R. Thomas

It is impossible to overestimate the crisis, fear, pain, and rage the survivor of sexual assault experiences after an attack. Add to that horrific mix the threat of HIV infection and you have a formidable recovery process. The advocate for the survivor of a sexual assault has a responsibility to assist in these related crises. Both involve counseling, crisis intervention, and education. Education about HIV/AIDS for the survivor of sexual assault must include an understanding of the Rape Trauma Syndrome, the unique learning and teaching opportunities presented by the services of a rape crisis program, and the societal stigma attached to both sexual assault and HIV/AIDS.

This chapter represents the lessons and experiences of one metropolitan agency, the Houston Area Women's Center, which provides counseling, education, and other services to victims of sexual assault. The Houston Area Women's Center provides shelter and support services to male and female survivors of sexual assault and of domestic violence. A common misconception about rape is that it is an act in which male perpetrators victimize female victims. In fact, both males and females rape and both males and females can be raped. For the purposes of this article, however, the pronoun "she" will be used when referring to the survivor, since statistics do show that more women than men are victims.

The Houston Area Women's Center conducts services based on a feminist approach. A fundamental premise of the feminist philosophy is that violence against women is not described solely by an individual woman being beaten by a spouse or being raped by a date during her first year in a university. Instead, these situations are descriptive of a societal assumption that women are less valuable than men and are not as deserving or capable as men to enjoy fully developed human identities. Since society constantly calls women's value into question, systematic violence against women is acceptable.

The feminist approach to the delivery of services for a survivor includes affirmation of the premise that her response to this violence is an adaptive survival response and not a unique, isolated pathological response. There are identifiable steps in the recovery from sexual assault—toward a path of independence, safety, and the pursuit of self-realization. Information, education, and support from those who have a clear understanding of the violent experience serve as catalysts toward recovery.

Through the feminist approach, advocates affirm the right of an individual to make her own decisions. The role of the advocate is to offer information that will foster informed decisions. Advocates seek to be ready with facts and concerns which are as clear and correct as possible. Unless there is a possibility of the survivor hurting herself or others, decisions made by the survivor are respected by the advocate.

Education cannot be conducted in a vacuum; there must be a consideration of the immediate state of the learner, which may affect the retention of the information, the logical format of the exchange of information (Is it verbal, a small brochure, a manual, a poster, a billboard?), and the environment in which the exchange of information occurs. For these reasons, the "teachable moment" for the survivor of a sexual assault and her friends and family will be discussed in this chapter across the dimensions of service delivery and of stages of recovery.

STAGES OF RECOVERY FOR THE
SURVIVOR OF SEXUAL ASSAULT

The recovery for the survivor of sexual assault is, unfortunately, not analogous to the recovery from a common physical laceration— bleeding and pain, eventual healing, and the possibility of a scar. The survivor of a sexual assault will experience a recovery that is "spiral" or "cyclical" in nature. The survivor will go in and out of crisis over a long period, experiencing distressing and repetitive symptoms. She will mentally and sometimes physically relive the rape, experience fear of seeing the assailant, as well as experience acute fear of another attack.

The Rape Trauma Syndrome is the cluster of symptoms often experienced by the sexual assault survivor. The syndrome has two phases: (1) the immediate or acute phase, in which the survivor has been thrown completely into crisis (disorganization), and (2) the long-term process of adjusting physically, emotionally, and cognitively to this life-shattering event (reorganization).

The crisis of the acute phase can last several hours or days. The reorganization phase can last for the rest of the survivor's life; not for a neatly plottable period after the sexual assault. A complete recovery back to the preexisting mental, physical, or emotional condition is impossible. The survivor has changed forever.

It is also important to note that crisis is not an emotional state limited to the initial disorganization stage. A variety of emotional triggers such as sights, sounds, feelings, or smells can send the survivor reeling back into disorganization. Crisis will often recur in the reorganization stage with no warning, such as when a survivor sees a car similar to the one in which she was sexually assaulted, or experiences an odor similar to the one prevalent during her assault.

In the long-term reorganization process, the survivor will experience distress or change in her physical, psychological, social, and sexual life. Physically, she may experience gastrointestinal distress, "body memory" related symptoms such as unexplained body soreness, or a perception of pain that does not respond to medication nor seem to diminish over time. Psychologically, she may have difficulty with negative repetitive thoughts, traumatic dreams, and a profoundly affected self-image.

Socially, she may respond to her assault by either choosing isolation or choosing never to be alone—sometimes even to a phobic degree. Sexual functioning can sometimes be the most affected area of a survivor's life, either diminishing drastically due to a survivor's disgust and fear of any sexual act, or increasing significantly—or perhaps even both.

The reorganization stage is the time when the survivor begins to take control of her life. Clearly, there are some ways to establish this control that are more beneficial than others. Adopting a life-inhibiting shame and guilt is one way to deal with sexual assault; understanding that the sexual assault was an act of violence purely based on the motivations of another may be a better way. Refusing to test for HIV because of a fear-induced paralysis is one way; taking control away from the perpetrator by actively facing an HIV test is another.

HIV/AIDS education for the survivor must include a consideration of her standing in the stages of recovery. Some services offered by women's centers will more frequently serve the survivor in the disorganization stage while others may be more attractive to a survivor who is reorganizing and ready to "get to work" on practical solutions. In addition to services, the format of education must be tailored with some knowledge and understanding of phases of recovery. A rape crisis program may choose to produce a recovery manual—a printed book that addresses crisis effectively but also discusses the resources needed once the survivor is ready to take control.

Perhaps most important, the critical point to consider is that not only does the survivor in crisis fail to understand fully what has happened to her, but she also does not anticipate fully the issues that may surface later. Experts in rape crisis programs have the ability to chart common concerns, fears, and reactions, including those related to the risks of HIV and AIDS. Materials and protocols can be developed that will assist when these issues are present, and the survivor or the friends and family can reorganize with clear and correct information.

SERVICES OF A RAPE CRISIS PROGRAM

All rape crisis programs are unique and do not necessarily offer the same services. However, many offer some or all of the following: (1) personal accompaniment volunteers, (2) a crisis hotline, (3) one-on-one counseling, and (4) peer-group support counseling. Volunteers who enter training for a rape crisis program can be trained to deliver all of these services, but many often choose to volunteer in only one or two. The multidimensional nature of services in a rape crisis program is designed for the nonlinear nature of a survivor's recovery from a sexual assault. These services, by definition offered on a "drop-in/drop-out" basis, are designed to require a minimum of preparation, paperwork, research, or structure on the part of the survivor. The services are designed to be accessible to the survivor in crisis, whether in the emergency room after the assault or ten years later after a nightmare about the assault.

A brief look at the services begins with a description of the personal accompaniment volunteer (PAV). When a survivor of sexual assault reports to law enforcement or to a medical facility, a protocol of evidence collection will be performed, called a "rape kit." In the best of circumstances, a specially trained physician or a Sexual Assault Nurse Examiner (SANE) will perform this protocol. Included in the series of medical and educational procedures is the careful removal of clothing over a large piece of paper in order to catch any bits of hair, flesh, blood, or other objects that may prove to be critical to the police investigation; the careful collection of any material under the nails; vaginal, oral, and rectal swabs; the testing for sexually transmitted diseases (except for HIV); and hair samples. While the protocols related to forensic collection are being performed, so also are other protocols on education for sexually transmitted diseases, for the risk of pregnancy for the female survivor, and for the possible side effects of any drugs administered. These are all performed by the health-care provider.

The PAV is present to help the survivor and her friends and family understand the often uncomfortable rape kit procedures and to advocate for the survivor, especially if faced with insensitive medical or law enforcement personnel; or even with insensitive friends and families. As with all services offered, the PAV services can be accepted or denied by the survivor or the friends and family members.

Experience shows that the majority of survivors communicate anxiety about HIV transmission during this visit with the health-care provider and the PAV. This is an opportunity for education on the human immunodeficiency virus, its transmission, and AIDS. However, since most survivors are in the "acute" phase of recovery at this point—in a state of disorganization and crisis—they will not be able to retain much of the information offered. For this reason, the PAVs may be trained and encouraged to give the survivor some form of written information to which she can refer later. In all instances, the hotline number is stressed, so that if the survivor is in a state of confusion or acute depression and cannot wade through the paraphernalia given to her at the hospital, she can call the hotline and have it explained to her again. The format of this education should be both written and verbal, with an emphasis on simplicity and action to be taken by the learner at another time.

This is a critical moment to provide education not only for the survivor, but also for the friends and family members who may be present. Because the sexual assault will have an effect on all those close to her, education on a variety of issues, including the HIV transmission risk, should be available for everyone. The PAV may be trained to speak to the friends and families about the risk of HIV transmission, about safe-sex practices, about availability and ethical issues related to HIV testing, and about the services available to them through a women's center or rape crisis program.

A "hotline" is a twenty-four-hour counseling phone service available through many rape crisis centers. Once again, due to the spiral nature of the recovery and because of the highly correlated anxiety and depressive reactions to a sexual assault, this service is designed to present a minimal obstruction to usage by the survivor. Hotlines are answered seven days a week and often have telephone numbers that are easy to remember. Volunteers estimate that fully half of the calls involve some question or stated anxiety about HIV. The inter- esting and commonly shared opinion by the advocates who fill hotline shifts is that it is incorrect to assume a correlation between testing for HIV and for anxiety about HIV. Logically, one might guess that once the testing has been done and the survivor has come up seronegative, anxiety would end about the "HIV piece." Instead, survivors in crisis sometimes doubt the results of the test and con- tinue to believe that they are at an extreme risk of having contracted HIV through the sexual assault. In counseling this survivor, as with counseling and advocating for any survivor, the advocate should stress education about potential risks as well as about available re- sources. What steps can the survivor take to allay some of her fears? Would she like the numbers of some resources for testing? The HIV- related fear is a manifestation of the control the rapist is continuing to have on the survivor. What steps can the survivor take in order to regain control?

One-on-one counseling and peer-group support counseling are offered by many rape crisis programs, but the one-on-one counsel- ing is usually only offered on a client-requested basis. One of the most common reactions to a sexual assault is a perceived state of extreme isolation. The survivor may believe that this is an experi- ence only she has had to live through, and that her reactions are unique and severely pathological. Peer-group support counseling is intended to normalize her reactions and to help her put her as- sault in a context of a sociological and political environment. The survivor's reactions are then identified as adaptive survival re- sponses as opposed to deviant or pathological. Most important, her assault is defined as the result of another's actions, and not in any way related to her own motivations or actions; in other words, it was not her fault.

For these reasons, the one-on-one counseling is often delivered on a request basis, while the peer-group support counseling is em- phasized by the advocates. In both the one-on-one counseling and peer-group support experience, HIV testing has often been com- pleted. However, this is an important opportunity to talk about re- sources for HIV testing, lowering the risk of transmission through safe-sex practices until the HIV test has been completed, and im- parting correct information about HIV and AIDS.

Peer-group support counseling is often structured for specialized populations. As an example, there may be a teen survivor group or an incest survivor group. Throughout the peer-group support environments, however, the issue of HIV and its transmission is reported by the facilitators of the groups as being an ongoing concern to the participants. Since peer-group support counseling is available to the client on a drop-in/drop-out basis (also called open groups), there are many different stages of recovery represented in a given group. Therefore, in almost every group experience, the facilitator will have the opportunity to talk about testing and education resources, discuss safe-sex practices, and address related anxieties. This is a critical opportunity for the learner to wrest control from the assailant by gaining information about sexual assault and the risk of HIV transmission.

TRAINING AND CONTINUING EDUCATION FOR ADVOCATES

Information on HIV must be correct, up to date, and imparted confidently by any educator, whether the educator or advocate is a staff member, a volunteer on the hotline, a PAV, or any person who comes into contact with the survivor. The latest medical information on HIV and AIDS comes fast and furious, however, and often in formats that are not "user-friendly" to those who have not received professional medical training. How can the rape crisis program most effectively keep their educators informed?

Rape crisis programs have intensive trainings that attempt to prepare the advocate to face the extremely complex web of issues the survivor will encounter. Part of the entry-level training for advocates may offer education on HIV and its transmission. In addition to the required entry training, a rape crisis program may wish to offer information through monthly mail-outs and quarterly or biannual professional inservices or meetings. Expert guest speakers may be asked to explain the latest developments in the medical community's understanding of risks of transmission and statistics on transmission to specialized populations.

Advocates must be cared for as well. An advocate who has pronounced anxiety surrounding the issue of HIV or AIDS will not be able to communicate effectively with the survivor about HIV. Through careful case management of advocates and by offering constant educational opportunities, this problem can be dealt with effectively.

It is extremely important that any information given about resources be updated carefully and systematically. The rape crisis program may desire to carefully screen their resources for hidden costs, for rude or insensitive personnel, or for unethical practices. In addition, a site visit can be made by the program's personnel or advocates in order to check facilities. Moreover, program personnel can provide education on sexual assault for their staff. For instance, if complaints are consistently lodged to the rape crisis program about an HIV testing resource that appears to be in a particularly dangerous area or in which the staff members are unpleasant, there should be careful consideration regarding whether to continue to refer clients to that facility. The consistency of trust in the services that a rape crisis program offers is the only real currency the program has to give to the community of survivors. Resources that do not serve the survivor destroy that trust.

ANONYMOUS VERSUS CONFIDENTIAL TESTING

There is a distinction to be made between referrals to anonymous versus confidential testing. This is of importance to the survivor of sexual assault because of the unique position this victim holds in the ranks of all victims of crimes.

The rape victim is the least believed victim of all of the violent crimes. This lack of confidence in the stories or testimonies of the survivors is illustrated by the questionable, possibly even immoral, practice of polygraphing rape victims. This practice is only systematically done with survivors of sexual assault. Robbery, burglary, assault, aggravated robbery—none of the victims of these crimes are asked to corroborate the experience of their victimization with a lie-detector test.

In addition, in the prosecution of a sexual assault case, the moral character of the victim is often called into question. Any evidence of behavior that might convince a jury that the victim is or was "promiscuous," used drugs or alcohol to excess, or was in any other way perceived of as low in moral character can be used by the defense to convince the jury that the sexual assault was consensual sex.

In an anonymous HIV testing environment, a patient is assigned a number. No other information is collected. There is no possibility of the information leaking to authorities or insurance companies, nor of it being subpoenaed. The sexual assault survivor faces monumental emotional problems in the months and years following the sexual assault. It would make her task of recovery even more difficult if she had to deal with her insurance company canceling her health or life insurance because of a seropositive result, or with a loss of a job because an employer discovered that a test was requested. The social and political tenor around HIV and AIDS is still permeated with misinformation, stigma, fear, and irrational acts of panic. The social and political tenor around sexual assault is, likewise, still permeated with misinformation, stigma, fear, and irrational acts of panic. This is the reality. The victim is protected from having the defense use the subpoenaed "confidential" results of an HIV test to prove consensual sex on the part of a "promiscuous" victim, or even the possibility of a lawsuit if there were transmission of the HIV virus from the victim to the assailant.

This ethical and resource issue of anonymous versus confidential testing should be carefully considered by a rape crisis program or in the design of services offered to the sexual assault survivor by some other agency.

CONCLUSION

The survivor of sexual assault who initiates contact with a rape crisis program has risked a tremendous amount of faith and trust. She has trusted that she will communicate to a stranger the most traumatic, embarrassing, shameful event of her life and that she will get an appropriate response. This is an absolutely critical moment, which may determine the survivor's access to services, advocates, and peers, and which may literally mean life or death for the survivor.

It is important to take into account a learner's readiness for information. There will be a teachable moment, dictated in some part by the stage of recovery from the sexual assault. Not only will the stage of recovery help to describe the learner's ability to retain information, but will also dictate the most effective format for the information.

The rape crisis program has a responsibility to impart information to the advocate and the survivor about HIV and AIDS in a factually correct and appropriate manner and can do so through a variety of services. Rape crisis programs may offer the one opportunity in a survivor's life to recover from a life-threatening event and to offer information that will insure her survival. There are a variety of practical and ethical considerations that must be taken into account by a rape crisis program or other agency that offers services to survivors in the design of its services to both survivors, their friends, and their families. HIV and AIDS adds a new and serious dimension to these practical and ethical issues.

12

Reaching In: The Challenge for HIV/AIDS Educators in the Criminal Justice System

James F. Duffield

BACKGROUND

In 1988, the report of the Presidential Commission on the Human Immunodeficiency Virus epidemic clearly recognized the importance of available HIV-related services, including health education programs, peer counseling, and other risk-reduction interventions. The report further underscored the important role community-based organizations play in getting educational messages to hard-to-reach populations. It particularly singled out the corrections system, strongly recommending a broad educational program for both inmates and staff. Several years later, the need for such programs continues to challenge HIV/AIDS service providers and educators as well as prison authorities and inmates.

In the United States, there are approximately 1.46 million men and women incarcerated in federal, state, and local correctional institutions (Osborne Association, 1995). While the number of inmates is 0.37 percent of the nation's population, those diagnosed with AIDS represent approximately 4.6 percent of the total number of cases reported in the United States (Hammett et al., 1994).

The incidence of AIDS in the prison population has been estimated at twenty times the rate in the population at large (Hammett, 1994). A study by the Centers for Disease Control in 1990 reported that, of the 65,171 inmates tested for HIV antibodies, 5.8 percent were positive (CDC, 1991). The findings of another study in 1991 put the rate of HIV seroprevalence in the U.S. correctional system in the range of 2 to 18 percent (Vlahov et al., 1991). In some states, this percentage hovers at the higher end of the spectrum. In New York, based on the rate of seroprevalence among new inmates, officials estimate that 11.5 percent of the men and more than 20 percent of the women in facilities operated by the Department of Correctional Services are infected with HIV (Hammett et al., 1994). This percentage rises in New York City jails, where rates of HIV infection run as high as 16 percent among men and 26 percent among women (Osborne Association, 1995).

An important consideration for HIV/AIDS service providers, medical staff, and educators is the significant rate of seroprevalence among people of color in the inmate population. In 1991, a survey of the state prison system demonstrated that, of those who underwent testing and reported the results, "3.7 percent of Hispanic inmates and 2.6 percent of Black inmates tested positive, compared with 1.1 percent of white inmates" (U.S. Department of Justice, 1993). Equally disturbing were the rates of infection found among Hispanic women "who, with a rate of 6.8 percent, were more than three times as likely as white women (1.9 percent) to be infected with HIV" (U.S. Department of Justice, 1993).

The prevalence of HIV infection in the prison system is all the more complex when one looks at the unique issue of incarcerated youth. In the general population, the Center for Disease Control reports that HIV infection in the thirteen to nineteen age group totaled 2,428 cases, through December 1994, in states with confidential reporting. The number of cases of HIV infection similarly reported for the twenty to twenty-nine-year-old cohort was 26,768 (CDC, 1994). While the rate of HIV infection among the general adolescent population may be relatively low compared to their older cohort, experience tells us that exposure and infection for the latter group, in all likelihood, occurred during their teen years—when sexual activity including prostitution, drug use and addiction, and homelessness add menacing elements of risk for infection for many youth.

These risks, however, do not get locked out when the convicted person is locked in. Sexual activities, whether coerced or not, and access to drugs are generally, if not officially, recognized to be realities of prison life. The corrections system, however, has traditionally "been reluctant to address issues related to drug use and sex in prison because . . . [it] believes that the frank discussion of these issues will undermine prison security by encouraging illicit behavior" (Smith and Dailard, 1994). This attitude has presented obstacles in the struggle to stem the tide of HIV infection in the prison system and extends the continuum of risk from the outside world through the prison walls, jail-house bars, and youth detention cells.

THE CORRECTIONS ENVIRONMENT VERSUS EDUCATION

Correctional facilities are, by their very nature, not caring communities. Rather, they are designed to confine and contain—not to nurture and attend to. The blueprint for a prison leaves little room for the ailing or the weak of body and mind.

The institutional culture of a correctional facility is one of homogeneity, conformity, and compliance. While this blanket of uniformity and control can occasionally become frayed from the resistance of individual inmates, the collective defiance of the prison population, or abuses by the system itself, with few exceptions the force of order remains intact.

Education, on the other hand, targets the individual as a member of a liberating social organization. It attempts to tap personal skills and preferences in order to develop and enhance competency. Education also entails goals that are future oriented. These characteristics run counter to the philosophy of a correctional institution and the realities of prison life.

AIDS also challenges the institutional philosophy and is viewed from the administrative perspective as a disruptive element in the orderly operation of the facility. Other inmates also feel threatened by the presence of HIV, and their response to it is often based on a lack of information, long-held myths, and prejudices. Inversely, it is the experience of medical providers and AIDS educators that "inmates generally welcome the opportunity to learn about HIV transmission and its prevention" (Remick and Szebenyi, 1994). Some report that inmates "respond positively to the program . . . [and] that it is not uncommon to reach up to 90 percent of the inmate population even with HIV/AIDS education programs that are strictly voluntary" (New York State Department of Health, 1994).

Reaching into a prison population with an educational program is, consequently, a delicate process. It commands an agile diplomacy to balance the perceived needs of the inmates with the concerns of the administration and staff. Any program for inmates will flounder against unbeatable odds if the full cooperation and authorization of prison administrators and that of security guards, medical and support staff, and inmates themselves are not confidently secured.

Who can best negotiate this precarious middle ground and provide the level of reliable and consistent education that the prison population needs? Many prison systems include HIV/AIDS information as part of their screening process of new inmates. However, it is easily and understandably lost in the overload of procedural and regulatory information being disseminated during the prison orientation. Those facilities with ongoing HIV education programs face additional obstacles. The underlying distrust between prison staff and inmates carries over into the measure of credibility prisoners will invest in the information disseminated by prison authorities. Inmates have demonstrated this distrust, responding more positively to information received "from outside agencies such as AIDS service organizations and public health departments" (Greenspan, 1991). With the support of these outside agencies, peer educators have been found to be the most effective, "because they speak the same language and are aware of the types of risk behavior that take place in prison" (Greenspan, 1991).

NEW DIRECTIONS

Prison authorities essentially control the content and degree of information available to inmates. This control has also included a reluctance to allow the active and direct participation of the community in prison operations. Whether because of political and social pressure or an enlightened approach, community-based organizations are gradually gaining access to prison facilities and inaugurating educational programs. Simultaneously, inmates themselves have initiated educational and support groups which have come to be recognized and validated by prison authorities. It is this combination of community involvement and inmate activism that has set the direction for the development and maintenance of educational programs within the prison environment.

An example of an innovative and viable effort is the AIDS Counseling and Education (ACE) program at the Bedford Hills Correctional Facility for Women in New York State. ACE was initiated by a small group of inmates with four main goals in mind: "to save lives through preventing the spread of HIV; to create more humane conditions for those who are HIV positive; to give support and education to women with fears, questions, and needs related to AIDS; to act as a bridge to community groups to help women as they reenter the community" (Bethel, 1995). To achieve these objectives, they began meeting and collecting HIV/AIDS-related materials in order to educate themselves. They soon were viewed by their peers as sources of information, counseling, and support. Eventually, the success and further potential of the program led to state funding, which allowed them to bring in community participants. This helped to reinforce and stabilize their relationship with the administration and gave them access to the community's educational and organizational skills. ACE currently operates a wide range of educational, counseling, and advocacy programs, and the model has since been replicated in other facilities.

INNOVATION IN EDUCATION AND BEYOND

Whether an educational program is developed by the inmates themselves or is initiated by the facility or a community organization, experience in this epidemic has demonstrated that traditional approaches to service delivery, treatment, preventative measures, and education are not only unsatisfactory, but too often fail to meet needs and accomplish goals. HIV/AIDS education requires ongoing assessment as educators and staff developers determine that curricula need to be far more inclusive in content, flexible in presentation, and responsive to the diverse issues affecting the intended audience. Increasingly, and usually because of consumer pressure, the intended audience has taken a more proactive role in the development of curriculum content and methods.

Experience in the prison system has demonstrated that HIV/AIDS education must be more than just the dissemination of information. It has been observed among injecting drug users that, while many "have received basic information about AIDS and HIV infection, . . . there are indications that risk-associated behaviors in this population are not affected by information alone" (Miller et al., 1990). According to seasoned educators and counselors, inmates resist changing their high-risk behaviors, and the problem is exacerbated by the plethora of untruths and myths about HIV and AIDS that thrive in the prison system.

HIV/AIDS educators should be intimately allied to on-site drug treatment and counseling programs. On a firm basis of consistent, relevant, and accurate information, educators collaborate with treatment providers "to facilitate the target population's development of a sense of ownership [of their behaviors and attitudes] . . . to move from thinking to action, . . . [and] to change sexual conduct and drug-using practices" (Ephraim, 1992). This sense of personal responsibility embraces a personal obligation to the health and safety of friends, family, and loved ones. Equipped also with the means to develop and maintain self-esteem, inmates are more likely to take the steps necessary to protect themselves while incarcerated and to sustain this modified behavior when they return to their communities.

The content and format of any HIV/AIDS educational program also hinge on several other factors: the availability of current epidemiological, etiological, and behavioral information; the character of the target audience; the potential for behavioral change; the points of juncture (i.e., the circumstances of the contact between educator and audience); the collateral needs of the inmates; and the assurance of confidentiality. These are not exclusive factors. They overlap and mutually affect their respective features.

The HIV/AIDS educator has the responsibility to develop and maintain an updated core of epidemiological and clinical knowledge about all facets of HIV illness. This generally is assumed to include modes of transmission, behavioral risks, the process of HIV illness, clinical symptomatology, the psychosocial elements of illness and those specific to HIV infection, the processes of loss and bereavement, and the realities of social and political stigma associated with HIV/AIDS.

However, a basic AIDS 101 curriculum does not address all the needs of the prison population. It has been asserted that injection drug use is the leading risk factor for HIV infection in the U.S. prison and jail system. Of the 25 percent of all prisoners who admit using needles for drug injection, 50 percent report sharing needles (U.S. Department of Justice, 1993). These statistics command a broader, yet relevant and practical, curriculum. They also dictate that educators serve in several capacities if they are to assist inmates in the process of gaining information and taking the necessary steps to modify behaviors, prevent infection, or cope with their seropositive status. The educator may also function as a facilitator or resource to support groups and counseling activities in the institution. The educator, as advocate, has the responsibility to intercede with prison authorities in an effort to integrate the concepts of a harm-reduction model that will be as compatible as possible with the prison system's mandate of containment and control. Understandably, prison authorities and staff view harm-reduction efforts as incongruous with the very nature of a prison environment. It would also be little welcomed by legislators who set and finance the system's mandate. Prisons, however, have another responsibility, and that is the safety of the inmates under their control. Therefore, every attempt should be made to negotiate with and persuade authorities that, to infuse the system with the spirit, rationale, and goals of harm reduction, they would be fulfilling that responsibility without any measurable loss of authority.

It is equally critical that any HIV/AIDS education activity run in tandem with a drug treatment program, counseling, and psychological support services. Changing drug-use behavior does not occur with knowledge alone. It is a lifelong process that again begins with accepting responsibility for one's own actions and a respect for self and others. It is an effort that requires consistent support and reassessment.

HIV/AIDS educators are an important link in this process. They provide the initial information that sets the foundation upon which other support services can function as agents for change.

CULTURAL CONSIDERATIONS

Prison is a microcosmic reflection of the greater outside society, with all the shifting variables of personalities and the divergent distinctions defined by culture. Typically, the term "culture" is interchangeable with the notion of ethnicity. In a broader sense, culture encompasses a substantial number of elements that are frequently overlooked when cultural diversity is considered a critical ingredient in the development of a curriculum package. Factors such as gender and age, along with ethnicity, may come to mind more immediately than others such as religion, economic status, family makeup, sexual orientation and self-identification, support networks (e.g., family, friends, institutions), geographical background (e.g., rural, suburban, urban), past experience with the criminal justice system, and identification with various subcultures (e.g., social, political, economic).

The educator's target audience consists of many overlapping bull's-eyes. This diversity is an important consideration. If it is neglected, the content and objectives of the curriculum will be off the mark in light of the life experiences of the intended audience. HIV/AIDS educators need to evaluate the broad cultural make-up of their target group and design a curriculum that is culturally relevant. With a diverse audience, the task of developing such a curriculum is an extensive task and, due to any number of restraints, may not be formerly realized. Consequently, the content and format must be so designed that they are flexible and create an open-ended atmosphere which allows the participants to freely comment on and challenge issues that they perceive as irrelevant and contradictory to their experiences. Failure to do this can leave the audience feeling disconnected and alienated. Any discussion on the risks of unprotected sex can be inconsequential, if not threatening, to a woman who will face a domestic situation where she does not have any latitude to negotiate sexual activity with her partner. Likewise, a dialogue on risk-reduction options for gay men will be viewed as irrelevant to men who have sex with men but who do not self-identify as gay. These are samples of the broader cultural considerations that educators must address in any HIV/AIDS curriculum.

Educators should not be completely satisfied with just attaining a level of cultural sensitivity. Recognizing the existence of differences and developing a respect for humanity's rich variations are only the initial steps toward cultivating a measure of cultural competency. It is here that the educator seeks explanations for behaviors and attitudes that are grounded in cultural experiences, validates those experiences, and collaborates with the participants in identifying culturally relevant and personally acceptable options.

A curriculum must also be couched in appropriate language. The educator should be able to communicate in a language that is both accurate and understandable. This not only makes the content comprehensible to the audience, but also avoids the pitfalls of idioms, slang, and euphemisms which vary by community and social subgroup. Appropriateness of language extends to written materials. They should be simply worded, explicit, and accurate in order to reach a maximum audience. Materials should not merely be translated into other languages; they should be *created* in those languages to ensure clarity and accuracy.

A goal of any HIV/AIDS education program is behavioral change through a process of knowledge, skill enhancement, and self-empowerment. However, this process has been developed almost exclusively for the outside world. In a correctional culture, the parameters of behavior are preordained, restrictive, and rigid. Behavioral changes directed at minimizing the risks for HIV infection hinge on the flexibility of options and the availability of the means to adopt those options. Whether certain behaviors, such as drug use and sexual activity, are routinely and consistently repressed, consciously ignored, or benignly tolerated, they are still prohibited behaviors. Nonetheless, they invariably occur and continue to put the participants at risk of infection unless they can take steps to protect themselves. If these behaviors are prohibited, "then the provision of information about safer-sex guidelines and contraception may be seen as unnecessary and may be denied" (Remick and Szebenyi, 1994). The barriers to information are even stronger when it comes to precautions for safer drug use. On a practical level, the reluctance to allow dissemination of information carries with it a denial of access to the tools of prevention (i.e., condoms and sterile needles).

This situation holds critical consequences for HIV/AIDS educators. The impact of the regulations that permeate the criminal justice environment is an important and unavoidable factor in creating a HIV/AIDS educational curriculum. The governance of these regulations becomes singularly significant when the conventional methods for reducing the risks for infection are unauthorized and prohibited and could put the inmate in jeopardy. Educators cannot rely on traditional recommendations for safer behaviors. Alternative approaches need to be developed that will prepare and equip inmates with the knowledge, self-esteem, self-empowerment, and supportive services to take practical and viable steps for protection. Again, the concepts of ownership, responsibility, and respect for self and others help create the basis for change.

JUNCTURES FOR CONTACT

The criminal justice system provides HIV/AIDS educators with a series of potential junctures where information and counseling can be accomplished. These points of contact dictate the extent of the educational activity. The educator must tailor the content and format to correspond to the fixed framework at any one of those junctures.

From the moment of arrest and detention, through the court process, and during the period of incarceration, the system is afforded opportunities to appraise detainees of various rules and regulations. These are the junctures that can also accommodate HIV/AIDS educational activities. Defined by the point of contact, the format and content may only consist of distributing written materials. It may allow for brief counseling or group orientation. While the period of final incarceration permits more extensive and substantive educational projects, it is not necessarily a stable span of time. Inmates may be moved to another part of the facility, where access is more limited, or they may be transferred to another facility altogether. For many inmates, their prison term may be relatively short. For example, in New York State, "the average inmate leaves the system after only 17 months and the turnover is 50% per year" (Remick and Szebenyi, 1994). This severely hinders any consistency and continuity in the educational process, and every effort should be made to link inmates to other available programs within the system or to outside service agencies.

The role of HIV/AIDS educators can extend to the post-incarceration period, when probation or parole set the parameters of the former inmate's release. As in the prison environment, it is critical that probation and parole officers also receive the information necessary to enable them to work with and counsel their clients. Familiarity with the physical and psychological impact of HIV illness will better prepare them to understand and accommodate. It is also critical that officers be aware of the availability of HIV/AIDS community resources that can supplement their own assortment of more generic service programs.

The period of probation or parole also gives educators the opportunity to provide a continuum of support and counseling to former inmates through linkages to community-based programs. The difficulty of the linkage and referral process is often a geographical one. Many inmates, upon release, will not be residing in a community near the facility where they were incarcerated. In some instances, they may be returning to a different state. Knowledge about coalitions or coordinating organizations in various areas can facilitate a linkage with community programs.

COLLATERAL ISSUES

Essentially, HIV/AIDS education aims to assist inmates in dealing with their serostatus. Optimally, the uninfected will be able to take steps to maintain their status, while those who are HIV positive will be better equipped to cope with their diagnosis. Achievement of these goals, however, does not complete the picture. It should be anticipated that the role of educators during the inmates' incarceration and the period of probation and parole will be perceived as that of advocate and liaison. Inmates, whether they are HIV positive or not, have many other concerns which the educator will, in all probability, have to address. Certainly, among these will be other health-related concerns, prison procedures, and questions relating to probation and parole and other personal issues. For many HIV positive inmates, their serostatus is not their priority. Concerns about families, legal questions, and plans for the future (jobs, housing, services, benefits) are foremost in their minds. These are the issues of survival, and educators will need to address them in order to maintain a level of credibility and relevance. The prison administration and on-site medical and social service staff represent an invaluable resource to address the varied issues raised by the inmates. This can also put the educator into the position of negotiator, conveying the concerns and views of the inmates to the prison staff.

Along with facilitator and negotiator, the educator invariably becomes involved in the role of discharge planner. As a liaison between the inmates and the community, and with the sanction of the administration, the educator can be instrumental in linking inmates with services and programs in the community that will assist in accessing benefits, health care, housing, drug treatment, and the like. Programs have been specifically developed to act, in part, as a "bridge" between the institution and the outside world. The AIDS in Prison Project of the Osborne Association in New York City provides information, counseling, medical advocacy, and service referrals through its HIV/AIDS clearinghouse and hotline. Some community programs have begun developing housing for former prisoners. This not only contributes to a stabilizing transition, but also ensures and facilitates access to services and a continuation of the educational and counseling process.

CONFIDENTIALITY

An overriding consideration for the HIV/AIDS educator in a prison environment is the element of confidentiality. In any congregate situation, privacy is a very thin veil. It is a very problematic issue for inmates and one that is vital to the success of any HIV/AIDS education effort. The stigma attached to HIV and the fears it raises in a contained prison society are critical deterrents to inmates seeking out HIV/AIDS counseling and other services. If a prison is designed to contain and control, the practical way to achieve these ends, aside from the walls and bars, is observation and scrutiny. In regulated societies, the rights of the individual are usually displaced and subsumed by the perceived greater need. In this environment, confidentiality implies exceptional treatment and runs counter to the institution's policy of uniform behavior.

This absence of privacy also extends to the exchanges and relations among inmates. The fear, whether real or imagined, of discovery, rejection, and reprisal prevent many inmates from taking advantage of HIV/AIDS-related counseling, education, and other services. Attempts to mask the HIV/AIDS component of an in-house program through the use of vague program labels or coy acronyms are euphemistic gimmicks that are rarely successful and usually counterproductive. Predictably, in a closed prison society, the fiction will be exposed and the true nature of a program will be disclosed. Disguising the real purpose of a program also makes recruitment of participants most difficult. The HIV/AIDS educator has few options to counter this situation. A fundamental technique is a contract, subscribed to by all program participants, that commits them to safeguarding each other's confidentiality and the integrity of the program.

With regard to prison personnel, educators have their own training skills and powers of persuasion to rely on. Prison staff need to recognize that the responsibilities of their profession do not preclude a basic respect for the individual, including regard for a fundamental right to privacy which does not automatically run counter to the mandates of the prison system.

It is important to note that the education and training of prison personnel is not limited to promoting the premise of an inmate's right to privacy. The overall success of any educational project requires the support of all levels of staff. If understanding comes from knowledge and is a foundation for support, then HIV/AIDS educators must also focus their energies on the prison staff. Addressing their concerns, countering misinformation with facts, and exploring the biopsychosocial aspects of HIV illness in a sharing and nonintimidating atmosphere can potentially validate staff professionalism, increase awareness to issues, and begin the process of enlisting staff support.

Interestingly, in cases where inmates are eager for HIV-related information, prison personnel are often suspicious of such programs because they see HIV/AIDS as an inmate problem and not one to be perceived as a personal issue. They also distrust these programs because they feel that they are not getting the complete story, but rather are being lulled into a false sense of security. Prison personnel need to recognize that HIV/AIDS education is a process that is beneficial to both themselves and the inmates.

CONCLUSION

Educators have few opportunities to reach so large and diverse an audience as they do in the prison system. Availability, however, is probably the only advantage. Accessing this audience calls for skill and diplomacy in fashioning a foundation of constructive and non-threatening trust with the prison administrators, security guards, prison support staff, and the inmates themselves. This relationship, however, will face many hurdles in an ongoing process of reaffirmation and validation.

Once trust is secured, the process of developing an appropriate and relevant curriculum begins. Some observers of the AIDS epidemic comment on the seemingly unprecedented involvement of persons living with HIV/AIDS in the planning and development of the very services of which they will also be recipients. This is not such a revolutionary concept. The old social-work maxim—"start where the client is"—implied the need for a collaborative relationship between provider and consumer. AIDS activists have embraced this counsel and given it new vitality and viability. HIV/AIDS education in the prison system, as elsewhere, is an equally fertile territory, that can generate a successful harvest through the proactive involvement of the inmates. It is the audience's self-perceived needs that determine and define the educators' strategies. The diversity of the audience also dictates that the educator choose not one strategy but, rather, an arsenal must be developed to address the varied concerns of the inmates coupled with their distinct personal and cultural experiences.

Educators must direct their efforts toward three distinct target groups: prison personnel whose understanding and support are absolutely necessary for a program to succeed, the inmate population for whom information is the first step toward survival, and peer educators who can provide trusted and insightful instruction and counseling.

At this point in the epidemic, prevention efforts are being reassessed for appropriateness and effectiveness. Until there are universal and unfailing methods of protection and the means for a cure, the conflict will be fought, in large measure, on the prevention front. HIV/AIDS educators must continue to take the lead in this, armed with accurate and relevant information and practical and effective strategies for prevention.

REFERENCES

Bethel, E. Rauh, ed. (1995). *AIDS: Readings on a Global Crisis*. Needham Heights, Mass.: Allyn and Bacon.
Centers for Disease Control (CDC). (1991). Publicly Funded HIV Counseling and Testing, United States, 1990. *Morbidity and Mortality Weekly Report* 40: 666–669.
Centers for Disease Control (CDC). (1994). HIV Infection Cases by Sex, Age at Diagnosis and Race/Ethnicity. *HIV/AIDS Surveillance Report* 6(2): 34.
Ephraim, J. C. (1992). "Developing an STD and HIV/AIDS Program for the Incarcerated Population." Workshop excerpts from the National Skills Building Conference, Washington, D.C.
Greenspan, J. (1991). AIDS in Prison: The National Perspective. *California AIDS Clearinghouse Reviewer* 3(1): 4.
Hammett, T. M., L. Harrold, M. Gross, and J. Epstein. (1994). 1992 Update: HIV/AIDS in Correctional Facilities. Washington, D.C.: U.S. Department of Justice, National Institute of Justice, pp. 14–18.
Miller, H., C. Turner, and L. Moses, eds. (1990). *AIDS: The Second Decade*. Washington, D.C.: National Academy Press.
New York State Department of Health. (April 1994). Criminal Justice Initiative Prison Program. Focus on AIDS in New York State. Albany, N.Y.: New York State Department of Health.
Osborne Association. (1995). "Aids in Prison Project Fact Sheet." New York: Osborne Association.

Remick, S., and S. Szebenyi. (1994). The Primary Care of HIV Infection in a Correctional-Facility Setting. *The AIDS Reader* 4(3): 79.

Smith, B., and C. Dailard. (1994). Female Prisoners and AIDS: On the Margins of Public Health and Social Justice. *AIDS and Public Policy* 9(2): 811.

U.S. Department of Justice. (1993). *Survey of State Prison Inmates, 1991*. Washington, D.C.: Bureau of Justice Statistics.

Vlahov, D., F. Brewer, and K. Castro. (1991). Prevalence of Antibody to HIV-1 among Entrants to U.S. Correctional Facilities. *Journal of the American Medical Association* 265: 1129–1132.

13

MAESTRO: A Cross-Cultural HIV/AIDS Training Curriculum for Diverse Disciplines and Communities

Chris Sandoval

As a Latino male, I have been fortunate to have a number of people in my life who have served as "maestros" (teachers); and, as is common in my culture, many of these teachers have been women. My grandmother and my mother were my spiritual teachers and taught me the importance of relationships, both familial and community-wide. They also helped me develop a world view that focused on "we" rather than "I"; one that stressed the importance of the group over the individual. Through their guidance, I have learned there are many pathways to knowledge and understanding, and it was their voices that I heard while trying to develop the following multicultural and cross-cultural training curriculum.

Training is both an art and a science, innate and learned, inherited and created. In nature, we see animals teach their young to hunt, to swim, and to survive the elements. In antiquity, our ancient parents taught their offspring their craft, their celebration of cultural rites of passage, and the technology of their times. In our modern day, training comes from multiple sources, which include, but are not limited to, the family, academic settings, religious institutions, and workplace environments. Training in the 1990s has undergone an evolution of revolutions of galactic proportions. We have experienced the peak performance (high technology) model that landed Apollo 11 on the surface of the moon. We have come to recognize life experience as a credible source of teaching through the use of peer counseling and education models.

We are now in the era of issue-specific trainings ranging from organizational development to sexual harassment in the workplace to specific health challenges to society like tobacco control, environmental health, and sexually transmitted diseases. And faced with a virus that can, at this time, only be defeated through widespread behavior change that must occur in increasingly diverse communities, the MAESTRO cross-cultural training model described in this chapter was developed.

Perhaps the greatest catalyst for change in the ways we teach an understanding, skill, and experience is cross-cultural AIDS training, because it forces us to reexamine our assumptions of the prevailing "way of doing business." Cross-cultural AIDS training for AIDS service providers is a process that consists of a series of action steps that promote proficiency in the understanding, skill, or experience of an individual or group to work with diverse cultural communities. Each of these proficiencies will be discussed in some detail.

PROFICIENCY IN UNDERSTANDING

The flawed Hubble telescope effect can create a cultural crisis that has a profound and sometimes irreversible effect. In the early days of the epidemic, at the AIDS ward in San Francisco General Hospital as Deputy Director of the Shanti Project and provider of one of the first peer-support service programs, I encountered several situations gone awry. In the first case, an African-American man with a Pentecostal upbringing began to pray aloud in the spirit. He was promptly sedated by an RN who thought he was hallucinating and becoming violent. In another case, a Japanese man with a strong Buddhist tradition indicated to his physician that he accepted his impending death as a natural process and was open to the experience. The doctor quickly made a psychiatric referral indicating that the patient was experiencing suicidal ideation and that a suicide watch was indicated. And still one more example—a counselor on staff came to me saying that the Latino client with the statue of the Virgin of Guadalupe had lit a votive candle, and was murmuring sounds under his breath while he held on to a beaded necklace. He stated, "That patient is really strange, it's like voodoo with all that stuff on his dresser." I had to explain that that was part of his spiritual tradition and that voodoo is also a spiritual practice in its own right.

Proficiency in understanding has enormous challenges for the HIV/AIDS prevention–education trainer. The increasing diversity of culture, the divergence of discipline or professional training background, and increasing mobility of society serve to complicate an already complicated communication environment. Some of the cross-cultural communication issues include the following:

1. Understanding the need to avoid technical language dialects associated with different disciplines, sometimes referred to as jargon.
2. Developing an awareness of the linguistic language dialects within monolingual communities, whether they are English, Spanish, or any other primary language group.
3. Recognizing and understanding body language communication dialects and styles.
4. Understanding communication mediums for cultural communities that value and utilize oral and visual traditions as the primary method of communication.
5. Establishing a universal communication dialect that speaks to people across different cultural experiences.

PROFICIENCY IN SKILL BUILDING

Proficiency in skill building for educating diverse communities is usually dependent on understanding both cultural common denominators that span all communities and cultural numerators that speak to cultural differences in specific communities. Invariably, you will find some diversity trainers who stress difference while others stress sameness when, in reality, the paradoxical truth is that both exist side by side. The challenge for educators is to establish terminology across cultures and disciplines to create an understanding that is cross-cultural and at the same time universal.

It is profoundly important to define culture before we begin our discussion on how to manage it. There are two fundamental truths about culture. First, it is the framework of every human being on the planet and second, culture is *more than ethnicity*. American history texts speak eloquently to the civil rights struggles of many disenfranchised communities, including ethnic–racial communities; women's communities; and lesbian, gay, bisexual, and transgender communities. Many cultural experts refer to this reality as the "social justice paradigm" of culture. However, culture is an all-embracing phenomenon that exists beyond race or national origin. Another way to view culture is to consider the building blocks that make up the cultural cathedral of mankind. Cultural difference is the root cause of many global conflicts, but conflict itself can be healthy because it provides opportunities for change. In fact, every breakthrough in human understanding has been preceded by a breakdown.

Culture is the blueprint of beliefs, behaviors, and identities which shape the perceptions of a person or a group of persons. It is an inheritance of ideas, practices, and attitudes which are conveyed and reinforced from generation to generation through society's institutions, such as family, church, and community. Culture defines right and wrong, delineates assumptions and expectations, and ultimately describes our dreams and the meaning of life. Culture is humankind's changing response to its environment; its interior search for connection to creation; and its need to act, react, and interact with members of the same species.

Culture can be further distinguished by examining its three stages of development and the specific qualities of each stage. The three stages of development in culture include Stage I—Cultural Genesis; Stage II—Cultural Metamorphosis; and Stage III—Cultural Rites of Passage. Let us take a closer look at each stage.

Stage I—Cultural Genesis

Cultural Genesis consists of cultural genes that predetermine the innate qualities or social environments we are born into, and they usually are not subject to change. Ten general variables comprise cultural genesis:

1. Ethnicity
2. Race
3. Country of origin
4. Economic class
5. Spiritual orientation
6. Language spoken at home (speaking, writing capabilities)
7. Sexual or affectional orientation (lesbian, gay, bisexual, heterosexual)
8. Geographic environment (rural, suburban, urban; hot, cold, or mild climate; monocultural, multicultural)
9. Physial abilities and disabilities
10. Family experiences

Stage II—Cultural Metamorphosis

Cultural Metamorphosis consists of variables or qualities that have the ability to transform or change the individual. Another ten variables fall into this second stage:

1. Marital status
2. Parental status
3. Military experience
4. Work experience
5. Educational experience
6. Environmental experience
7. Religious experience
8. Civil rights experience
9. Income experience
10. Survivor experience

Stage III—Cultural Rites of Passage

Cultural rites of passage are qualities or variables that denote a common social group experience. Generally speaking, there are four cultural rites of passage:

1. Voluntary immigration
2. Involuntary immigration (flight because of war or famine or disaster)
3. Acculturation (length of stay in new area of residency)
4. Similar historical experience (the Holocaust, Vietnam, HIV disease, the civil rights movement, religious community).

PROFICIENCY OF EXPERIENCE

Proficiency of experience, or hands-on ableness to educate or deliver services to "hard-to-reach" or culturally different populations, is highly regarded and often difficult to acquire by agencies funded to serve them. Furthermore, both novice and experienced trainers encounter a number of barriers that can greatly impact their degree of success. Some of those barriers include the following:

Lack of Trust   AIDS activists have had a long-standing issue of trust with the institutions of government that were slow to respond to the advent of the AIDS epidemic; and, when they did, often responded slowly as bureaucracies tied up in their own red tape. For example, the Food and Drug Administration (FDA) was perceived to be unnecessarily slow in its authorization of experimental drugs that could provide some medicinal effect to a desperate population.

Lack of Relationship Although many individuals from faith communities were among the first to provide support to HIV infected people, many gay men of all colors had difficulty in accepting their help because many gay men lacked a relationship with religious institutions, which had judged their sexual orientation as sinful and unacceptable. Gay men who had left or been pushed from these institutions for decades now were left in a state of wonderment that many of these same institutions were now reaching out to them.

Historical Conflict White Americans and communities of color have had historical conflicts around issues of equity, parity, and equality. The HIV epidemic is simply one more context for the ongoing debate. For example, there have been, and continue to be, uneasy dialogues over funding priorities and the use of epidemiology to drive funding decisions.

Rapidly Changing and Evolving Environment In 1993, my agency undertook a three-part needs assessment of training and technical assistance (TAT) focused on the technical-assistance needs for education and prevention providers in California. We constructed a model of TAT and a curriculum called the "University Without Walls," only to find, six months later, that the results of the prior needs assessment did not match the current request for TAT by providers. It is clear that the HIV epidemic is in a rapidly changing and evolving environment.

Differences in Exposure to Training and Educational Paradigms An academic approach or a training curriculum generally has a specific discipline which serves as the framework for understanding and interpreting the information being presented. By its very nature, its emphasis is narrow and deep. That kind of focused, laser-quality emphasis has its advantages and its disadvantages. HIV disease has a severe need for specialized areas of expertise and yet, at the same time, demands comprehensive approaches to problem solving that utilize many disciplines to address problems. Case managers, for example, are routinely called upon to utilize a variety of disciplines and interact with a wide array of service providers in their efforts to secure needed client services over time. Such depth of knowledge continues to increase as our care system continues to be challenged by the disease.

Lack of Knowledge, Experience, or Information of the Cultural Community Being Served Interventions, approaches, and models of education and prevention need to reflect cultural relevancy and better serve diverse populations. Channels of credibility for a specific cultural group of emphasis change from community to community. The Hmong communities' most effective and credible teachers are not MPHs, outreach workers, or peer educators, but the shaman, who is the spiritual leader and teacher within that community. Native Americans' source of highest credibility is its medicine men. Meztec Indians "look" Mexican, speak Nahuatl and not Spanish, and work side by side with Spanish-speaking Mexican nationals as seasonal workers in the fields of California. The need to know the most effective messenger and the most effective vehicle for the message is paramount in stopping the spread of HIV disease and supporting the infected and their families.

Inability to Mediate Conflict Conflict in the AIDS epidemic has internal and external dimensions. Internal to many communities, the issues of power sharing between traditional gatekeepers from the first generation of caregivers and youthful newcomers have fueled public debate. External conflicts between gay white male AIDS activists and people of color activists over limited resources and power sharing have erupted into conflict that is at once both subtle and dramatic. Having mediators who can call conflicting parties back to the mission and to reasonable solutions that allow everyone to save face is critical.

Simply put, managing a multicultural, multidisciplinary staff in a motion-filled work environment creates chaos, conflict, organizational confusion, and growth. This is true for a kibbutz, a cloister, or a community-based organization.

GUIDELINES FOR AIDS PREVENTION CROSS-CULTURAL TRAINING

As previously stated, training workshop participants is both an art and a science. It requires the trainer to fall back on formal and informal training which he or she may have experienced, as well as to develop the skill to intuit and use human facilities which exist beyond the scope of human intellect. Trainers frequently fail to make the mark for a client because they utilize logic as the sole problem-solving approach when conflict and misunderstanding are frequently experienced in the psychological and sociological environments of human passion and emotion, rather than through cognition.

Training in a culturally diverse setting is a process best achieved through a structure. The following training guidelines will assure a lively, fun-filled, and nonthreatening training process built on a twenty-year career of in-service training for highly diverse community and private-sector environments. The seven steps in this process are discussed in greater detail in the remainder of this chapter.

1. Establishing ground rules for communication
2. Establishing a deeper understanding of who we are in the work-place, the home, and the community
3. Building trust and relationship
4. Revisiting the mission to review what it says and what it does not say
5. Naming and identifying the demons that haunt, perplex, and confuse a work environment
6. Developing an agency action agenda for meeting the needs of volunteers, clerical support staff, front-line practitioners, program managers, administrators, and board members
7. Taking the next good step

A STEP-BY-STEP VIEW OF THE TRAINING PROCESS

Step 1—Establishing Ground Rules for Communication

The objective of formulating ground rules is to provide a safe space in which participants feel safe to express concerns that emanate from fears, perceptions, or realities confronting members of a par-ticular group of individuals. It is important that participants recognize and internalize that, "It's OK to disagree, but it's not OK to disrespect someone with a differing viewpoint." I call this process, "respectful interaction."

On standard easel paper, write out the title "Ground Rules for Respectful Interaction" and list out a number of communication commandments. This exercise is done before any introductions or statement of purpose. It is critical to lay the ground rules before beginning the training process. I start by identifying the following seven ground rules.

Ground Rules for Respectful Interaction

1. Respect—in the spoken word, in vocal intonation, and in body language.
2. A person will hold the floor for no more than three minutes. No filibustering.
3. Raise your hand for recognition by the facilitator or trainer.
4. Speak one at a time. No cross talk or whispering.
5. No smoking.
6. Attentive active listening. Can we hear with eloquence?
7. What else should we include as ground rules for respectful interaction?

Step 2—Who Are We?

There are a number of interactive exercises that help participants get to know each other effectively. Convention, workplace limitations, and other parameters leave many wondering about their colleagues' life experiences and seeking a personal connection with coworkers. This particular exercise helps to answer everything "inquiring minds want to know." The name of the exercise is *Tú y Yo* (You and Me). The exercise begins by having the participants answer a list of questions (see Figure 13.1) on large pieces of butcher paper placed on the walls around the room. The facilitator then uses the rich information provided to make connections among the particpants and to highlight common cultural values, while still acknowledging and valuing any differences within the group.

Step 3—Building Trust and Relationship

Trust building takes time, usually over an extended period of interactive experience. Knowing people's boundaries and recognizing the triggers in the diplomatic minefield can be a useful beginning for a group of dissimilar people brought together to focus on a similar mission. The following exercise begins to look at those issues. The exercise is called *¡Ya Basta!* (Enough Is Enough!).

Eight people, representing two sides of an issue, organizational layer (management and labor), or cultural group of emphasis, are asked to form a fish bowl. A fish bowl is a small panel or group that is formed in the middle of a larger audience so that their behaviors and dialogue may be observed by the entire group. Each side is represented by four individuals. The facilitator then asks panel group one to complete the following statement:

In order to build trust and relationship with me, you must never, ever

_____

and you must always, always _____

to maintain that trust and relationship.

Then, the facilitator asks panel group two to also complete the same statement. The facilitator then helps the groups to see that both frequently have very similar responses, expectations, and boundaries.

Figure 13.1
"You and Me" Questions

1. The name people call me is:_____

   My name is: _____

2. Ethnicity (nationality or family ancestry):_____

3. Race (American Indian, African American, Asian/Pacific Islander, Communities of Mixed Heritage, European American, Latino, or ?)

   _____

4. Economic class raised in. My present economic class is (working class, blue collar, white collar, middle class, etc.):_____

   _____

5. Spiritual orientation raised in:_____

   My spiritual orientation is: _____

6. Languages spoken: _____

7. Sexual/affectional orientation: _____

8. Political orientation (liberal, moderate, conservative): _____

9. Marital status (single, married, widow/er, divorced, living with

   someone): _____

10. Parental status: _____

11. Military experience: _____

12. Profession/occupation/job title: _____

Step 4—Revisiting the Mission

In highly diverse environments, people frequently move to create gains for groups with which they identify. Many writers have referred to this phenomenon as "balkanization" of the workplace and of society. In general, people tend to advocate the agendas of specific groups with which they belong and identify. Using the agency's or organization's mission as a means of discussion or departure is a good way to avoid balkanization and, instead, gets people on a path of universal shared advocacy, creating equity, parity, and cultural democracy. I call this process "Revisiting the Mission." Here are several ways to begin the discussion.

Figure 13.1 (*continued*)

13. Educational experience: _____

14. Environment (urban, suburban, rural): _____

15. Role models: _____

16. Positive behaviors I role model for family and friends: _____

_____

17. Oppression experience: _____

18. Social justice issues most important to me (civil rights, women's rights, children's rights, the environment, etc.)

_____

19. Survivor experience (terminal illness, violence, divorce, etc.):

_____

20. Family generations in the United States: _____

21. My favorite color is: _____

22. My favorite food is: _____

23. My favorite dessert is: _____

24. A symbol that describes me is: _____

25. Three words I live by are: _____

1. Revisit the mission of the organization; review it, rewrite it, and use it as the primary vehicle to develop (or reflect on) goals and objectives for the organization and its bylaws.

2. Conduct a management audit that reviews job descriptions against the mission statement and the organizations's goals and objectives.

3. Create a strategic plan involving all the stakeholders of the organization with appropriate time lines and a delegation of responsibilities to the stakeholders and a commitment to implementation and evaluation.

4. Develop a code of ethics or operating principles with the stake-holders to emphasize "fairness" as a governing principle in the behaviors of all the stakeholders' interactions.

5. Develop a plan to support affirmation, recognition, and reward for the accomplishments of individuals who exceed strategic-planning goals and objectives. This is particularly useful in encouraging higher productivity and preventing burnout and disillusionment.

Step 5—Naming the Demons that Haunt, Perplex, and Confuse a Work Environment

Perhaps there is no greater problem than naming issues of con-flict or identifying the difficult personalities that continue to fo-ment unrest, lack of morale, and low productivity; especially if the people at the top of the organization are responsible for it. Consult-ants frequently get feedback that the "the emperor has no clothes," or that the "take no prisoners school of management" is the stan-dard operating procedure, but are afraid to report their findings since it is sometimes the client we are working for who is responsible, in some way, for supporting the problems that exist. A useful tool to naming the demons is something I call "evidence inventory," which helps to set the groundwork for data-driven decision making. The evidence inventory includes the following six workplace informa-tion documents:

1. Organizational flowchart
2. Breakdown of staff by gender, ethnicity, position, disability, sexual or affectional orientation, age, and other cultural variables
3. Secondary data sources, including historical documents like prior surveys, annual reports, case statements, governing docu-ments, and client feedback information, to name a few examples
4. Confidential focus groups' findings of key informants and stake-holder networks; the findings should not be attributed to any single person or group of persons by name
5. Market or behavioral research literature summaries that help to give us comparative data on similar organizations
6. Individual, confidential, and anonymous mechanisms for feed-back, like opening a channel for written communication through an ombudsman or committee to identify what works and what does not

The information for the evidence inventory should be gathered prior to the group meeting. This can be done by individuals or teams of people. The purpose of the inventory is to let the group meet and discuss what has been documented organizationally—to examine what information says (or does not say) about who the organization is and what it is about.

The results of the evidence inventory are then integrated into an agency report titled an "Agency Action Agenda."

Step 6—Agency Action Agenda

The Agency Action Agenda is the product of the training and technical assistance process that was undertaken in Steps 1 through 5. The table of contents for the Agency Action Agenda may look something like this:

Table of Contents

- Dedication page (a statement of vision which may be dedicated to a client, a hero or heroine in the community, or to the people we have lost in the epidemic)
- The agency, its mission, and its accomplishments
- Principles (or themes) for designing and delivering successful community programs
- State of the agency (findings of the evidence inventory and internal data collection)
- Recommendations for action (including time line and evaluation)
- Conclusion

Step 7—The Next Good Step

This step points to a number of potential possibilities. Undergoing an extensive training and technical-assistance process that documents need, recommendations, and an action agenda can be a thoroughly engrossing process that produces a ripple effect throughout the agency. There are a number of different strategies that should be undertaken during the process to secure a positive outcome. They include the following:

1. Develop a transition management plan
2. Document the training process
3. Incorporate training as an objective for managing change and as an ongoing organizational practice
4. Create training goals and objectives for the different organizational layers within the agency (e.g., the Board of Directors, the

Honorary or Fundraising Board, senior management, the middle or program management team, staff, clerical or administrative support staff, volunteers, consumers or clients, related agencies, the public at large, the media, and donors)

5. Establish ongoing feedback mechanisms, like quality circles, a conflict-mediation ombudsmen, confidential staff, and consumer surveys

6. Evaluate all program activities to see what works and what does not

7. Encourage trainings and technical assistance on improving reporting responsibilities and activities to funding sources

CONCLUSION

As the HIV/AIDS epidemic moves into the next century, perhaps the single greatest step that an agency that is serious about cultural diversity and saving lives can take is planning and implementing diversity trainings. Our ultimate mission is to stop the spread of HIV disease as well as to support people living with HIV disease, their significant others, and families. We must do so in a social environment whose only real common denominator is its diversity. Diversity, by its very nature, can be complex and it is further complicated by the impatience of an era where we communicate in sound bites and look for magic-bullet answers for many of our problems.

Managing rapid change in our knowledge, skill, and experience through ongoing training will be the difference in saving the lives of the uninfected and prolonging the lives of the infected. This global pandemic requires an aggressive community response in managing the local epidemics in all of our diverse communities. We must remember that cultural incompetence may put the innocent at risk for HIV disease and may hasten the death of our loved ones who are infected. We already know that cultural incompetence is the root cause of much conflict among those of us in the field of wellness. We know that it is the ongoing cause of racial strife and a major cause of human misery. We must come to realize that cultural incompetence coupled with the HIV pandemic is a certain formula for human suffering that can only be measured by grief and loss. MAESTRO, the foregoing cross-cultural HIV/AIDS training curriculum, begins to answer that challenge.

14

Effective Program Evaluation

Martin L. Forst and
Melinda K. Moore

Are AIDS educators making a difference in their efforts to prevent the transmission of HIV? Are some programs or strategies working better than others? Why? These are just some of the questions that evaluation efforts seek to address. We know that finding the answers is often difficult. Evaluation can be expensive, both in terms of dollars and human resources. But good evaluation is an essential part of any HIV/AIDS education and prevention program.

In many respects, evaluation can be viewed as an investment in the future. A disease like AIDS has such dire physical, social, economic, and political consequences that evaluation takes on special significance. The benefits of effective prevention programs are literally a matter of life and death. Therefore, it is imperative that we know now, and on a continuing basis, exactly what services we are delivering and to whom, what interventions are working with which target populations, and why.

Program evaluation is not meant to be punishment from the gods. Nor should it be considered only a necessary condition for securing program funding from a government agency. Evaluation is best viewed as an aide to program administrators. Evaluation can benefit AIDS education and prevention programs in two basic ways. Most important, an effective evaluation can improve program services and thus directly benefit your target population. Sound evaluation can also help your program receive additional funds—either through renewed funding from the original source or new funding to address unmet needs identified by the evaluation.

The evaluation of AIDS education and prevention programs presents a host of difficult problems. Following clients over time to determine if they have changed their behavior raises both practical and ethical issues. Even administering a simple knowledge-based test to hard-to-reach populations, such as injection drug users, can present almost insurmountable logistical difficulties.

Theoretical problems also exist when attempting to select the best model for designing and interpreting evaluation results. Yet the evaluation of AIDS education programs is essential if public-health planners and educators are to employ the most cost-effective strategies to stop the spread of HIV. The recent National Research Council report stresses this point:

Program evaluation in the context of AIDS prevention is as difficult as program implementation itself, and as necessary. . . . The panel believes that future AIDS prevention efforts should plan and allocate sufficient resources to obtain sound evidence about what works best to alter those behaviors that are known to transmit HIV. (National Academy of Sciences, 1991)

This chapter is geared to the achievement of practical yet effective program evaluation. The tips presented will not only help fulfill contractual requirements with your funding source, but help assess how well the program is serving your target population.

More generally, program evaluation will help determine what sorts of local education and prevention strategies are effective with different target populations. Attaining this level of evaluation would be quite an accomplishment; to date it has not been done well. As the National Research Council states, "Given their emphasis on service delivery, the community-based organization [CBO] projects that have been funded have not paid much attention to evaluation. . . . At present, none of the CBOs can demonstrate the effectiveness of the interventions they have implemented" (National Academy of Sciences, 1991).

It is important to realize from the outset that ideal evaluations are rarely possible to conduct. This is true for several critical reasons. First, the level of funding provided, particularly to local education and prevention programs, usually does not permit the devotion of adequate resources to evaluation. The old maxim, "you get what you pay for," is generally true in the field of evaluation. It is simply unrealistic to expect a thorough, sophisticated program evaluation for a few thousand dollars. Second, the nature of the target population may limit what an evaluation can accomplish. It is difficult at best to consistently measure changes in knowledge, attitudes, beliefs, and behaviors among, say, homeless and runaway teens in an urban setting.

The evaluation component of a grant application will increasingly become a critical factor of public funding in the future. It is, therefore, essential for local program managers to grasp fully the fundamentals of effective program evaluation. We want to reiterate that a good evaluation can improve program performance. And effective evaluations can be done if a few basic rules are followed. We start with basic definitions and concepts.

LEVELS OF EVALUATION

The term *evaluation* implies different things to different people. A recent report of the Committee on AIDS Research and the Behavioral, Social, and Statistical Sciences defines the scope of evaluation through a series of questions about a program or intervention: What was done? To whom, and how? What outcomes were observed? What do the outcomes mean?

Answering all these questions well in a local program evaluation is a tall order. Many things are not feasible in small-scale evaluations. For example, the National Research Council recommends "randomized field experiments" to evaluate AIDS education and prevention programs. But randomized field experiments are quite complicated and expensive, and not within the realm of possibility for programs without a sizeable evaluation budget.

Some parts of a program evaluation can be relatively easy, such as counting the number and types of clients your program reaches or carefully documenting what interventions you provide to different clients. Even doing these elementary tasks is more than many programs have done in the past. More sophisticated evaluations may try to assess levels of change among clients (e.g., increased knowledge about the transmission of HIV or decreased high-risk behaviors). Ultimately, the program evaluation is intended to determine if your program has reached its stated goals and objectives.

For some programs, all evaluation questions cannot be answered. It may be necessary to focus the evaluation on specific issues, just like it is necessary to focus (or target) the program itself. That is, you might have to be selective and concentrate on addressing specific questions, realizing that others may be beyond your capabilities. From the start of the program—even when it is in the planning stages—it is important to know your limitations as well as your capabilities.

TYPES OF EVALUATION

Over the years, much evaluation terminology has developed, some of which is jargon used only by evaluation practitioners. There remains confusion in terminology, even among experts in the field. In this chapter, we use the terminology adopted by the National Research Council for Evaluation of AIDS Programs.

The two main types are process and outcome evaluation. The process evaluation is designed to answer the following question: Is the program reaching its intended audience? In general, a process evaluation is easier to conduct, requiring less sophisticated design, methodology, and instruments. By contrast, an evaluation that attempts to assess the outcomes or effectiveness of an intervention, or an entire program, and what those outcomes mean is a more complicated endeavor. The outcome evaluation seeks to answer these questions: Is the program making a difference? What works better?

Both process and outcome evaluations are necessary because they are intimately connected. If the outcome evaluation tells you that your goals and objectives were achieved, the process evaluation will help tell you why. If your objectives were not met, the process evaluation will explain what went wrong.

Process Evaluation

Process evaluation initially addresses two broad questions: What was done, and to whom and how? The purpose of a process evaluation is to examine the linkages between inputs and outputs. The inputs are the human and material resources the program uses and the outputs are how those resources were used.

More specific process-evaluation questions concern whether the appropriate clients are being targeted, as well as whether all those in need are being reached. The process evaluation also addresses the organizational structure and management style used to implement the program. More specifically, a process evaluation attempts to answer the following questions:

1. Who are the clients in the program?
2. Are they the ones originally targeted by the program?
3. What proportion of those targeted are receiving program services?
4. Why did some of the target population not receive services?
5. How did the program's organizational structure affect the provision of services to clients?
6. What is the extent of agreement within the organization about the goals and objectives of the program?

7. What impact did the program staff's experience, education, and cultural background have on program implementation?

How human and material resources are put together to produce the outputs is critical to evaluation; they concern program implementation. When done properly, the process evaluation describes what aspects of the program were responsible for producing the observed outcomes.

It is important to realize that an evaluation can show that a program was a success or failure for several possible reasons. If the evaluation indicates that the program has failed, the program may have been based on an inappropriate theory, the program implementation may have been flawed, or the evaluation itself might have been designed poorly.

Process evaluations are generally less expensive to conduct than outcome evaluations. They can be done more readily by in-house staff at relatively minimal expense. Process evaluations can include direct observation of project activities, surveys of service providers or clients, and the review of program records.

Outcome Evaluation

Outcome evaluation is concerned with the accomplishments of a program relative to its goals and objectives. That is, this type of evaluation identifies the objectives of the program and its specific purposes, and through various methods, attempts to determine the extent to which the objectives have been achieved. The National Research Council states,

The purpose of outcome evaluation is to identify consequences and to establish that consequences are, indeed, attributable to a project. This type of evaluation answers the questions, "What outcomes were observed?" and, perhaps more importantly, "What do the outcomes mean?" (National Academy of Sciences, 1991)

Outcome evaluations tend to be the more expensive type of evaluation. Large program evaluations require a great deal of resources and money. The National Research Council concluded that "the cost of an outcome evaluation sometimes equals or even exceeds the cost of actual program delivery" (National Academy of Sciences, 1991).

There is some debate about how sophisticated outcome evaluations must be—particularly for local AIDS education and prevention programs. Some people contend that they must be complicated and sophisticated. To be done thoroughly, this is generally true. However, the degree of complexity and sophistication varies to the extent that the program goals and objectives are complicated.

When doing complex outcome evaluation, it is necessary to assume that there is a theory underlying the program. The evaluator should attempt to determine what theory is being used. The goal is to determine what happened to the clients after the theory was implemented, compared to what would have happened if the theory had not been implemented. In a sense, an outcome evaluation is a test of this theory. Program evaluation can thus be an important link between theory and practice. For example, the Health Belief Model holds that there is a relationship between knowledge, attitudes, and behavior. If your program embraces this model, the outcome evaluation should determine if program participants underwent significant changes in these domains as a result of your program.

A major difficulty of outcome evaluation is determining whether the outcomes are the result of the program's interventions, or of some other factors. To reach this conclusion with confidence, it would almost be necessary to create an artificial laboratory situation in which the program could control all variables. This "ideal" is often impossible in most program evaluations; each study is unique, and most social variables cannot be easily controlled. This is particularly true when working with hard-to-reach populations, such as migrant farm workers or Southeast-Asian refugees. However, even if attribution cannot be fully determined within a community-based evaluation setting, the information you *can* obtain makes the attempt well worth the effort.

UNDERSTANDING YOUR TARGET POPULATION

In order to serve your target populations well, it is necessary to "reach" them. Reaching them has two meanings: first, to physically locate them, and second, to communicate effectively with them.

Generally speaking, locating the target population is not the biggest obstacle in AIDS education programs, even for so-called hard-to-reach populations. In one statewide evaluation of California's AIDS education programs, almost all of the programs reached the designated number of their target populations (Moore and Forst, 1993). Of course, this is not always the case. Not everybody wants to be found. Some people, like gay-identified ethnic minorities, want to maintain anonymity; some people, like injection drug users, want to avoid contact with the legal system.

A greater problem faced by health educators is effectively communicating with the target population, once located. In order to communicate effectively, it is necessary to understand the target population—its values, attitudes, and culture. These more nebulous variables can, on the one hand, represent barriers to communication. But if the target population is well understood, these variables can also enhance opportunities for communication and eventual behavior change.

In the past, many health educators have stated that "health education is health education," insisting that health-related information is and should be delivered in a manner devoid of its cultural context. They have argued, for example, that the information needed to address HIV risk is straightforward and easily understood. These educators have tended to ignore or discount the cultural context in which health-related information must be delivered. However, providing (and evaluating) effective interventions requires not only delivering the correct and updated information; it also demands that the information be delivered in ways that the targeted population understands and accepts. Program administrators and evaluators must understand the cultural meaning derived by the target population from the information being imparted. And cultural meaning can be determined only by studying the target population or enlisting members of that group to participate in the design and delivery of the intervention. Understanding your target population can be accomplished in a variety of ways:

- Read about the target population
- Interview members of the target population
- Conduct an ethnography of the population
- Have a member of the target population on program staff

It is important to remember that no racial, ethnic, or cultural group is homogeneous. Within any racial, ethnic, or cultural group there are many subcultures, all with unique ways of communicating and behaving. Conducting mini-ethnographies can provide you with a way to learn about specific subcultures. A mini-ethnography would provide you information on how people behave, the "language" used by the group, what they believe to be important, their attitudes towards those outside the group, and so forth.

Ethnography can become a powerful tool in the hands of health educators—and evaluators. For example, if you are attempting to reach Latino injection drug users, you first need to understand that subculture. By sending someone to places where that target population congregates, over time, a skilled ethnographer can learn a great deal about this population, gaining information essential to planning an effective intervention.

SPECIFYING CLEAR GOALS

Carefully worded program goals are necessary for the selection of appropriate program objectives and, particularly, outcome measures to test the effectiveness of a program. Too frequently in the past, programs have been hampered by poorly written goals (i.e., goals that did not reflect desired outcomes).

Goals are general. The Centers for Disease Control's overall mission is to "prevent the spread of HIV infection." This is the "big picture." Local program goals should also be written with the broad stroke of a brush. A few examples of local program goals are as follows:

- "The goal of this program is to increase knowledge about HIV transmission routes among homeless and runaway teens."
- "The goal of this project is to change attitudes about condom usage among migrant farm workers." ·
- "The goal of this program is to improve safe sex negotiation skills among sex partners of injection drug users."
- "The goal of this project is to enhance safe substance use practices among injection drug users."

CRAFTING REALISTIC OBJECTIVES

Objectives are more specific than goals. They should be stated in a way that, if they were met, they would fulfill the program's general goals. Objectives should also be written in a way that would allow them to be measured—thus, they should be stated as "measurable objectives." As the National Research Council suggests,

In addition to the overarching goal of eliminating HIV transmission, the panel recommends that explicit objectives be written for each of the major intervention programs and that these objectives be framed as measurable biological, psychological, and behavioral outcomes. (National Academy of Sciences, 1991)

The wording of objectives is important. They should be written with the overall program evaluation in mind. For example, it is relatively difficult to measure change. It may not be wise to write an objective like, "the target population will increase knowledge of HIV transmission by 35 percent." With the objective stated this way, the evaluation requires a pre–post design. Unless you collect baseline data beforehand, you will have no basis of comparison—you will not be able to determine change.

If you have only one chance to educate the target population and one chance to measure knowledge and attitudes, it is best to write the objective in a different way. You could say, "the target population will attain a 90 percent competency level in knowledge of HIV transmission and prevention." So stated, you do not need to determine what the level of knowledge was before the program intervention.

One of the major difficulties encountered in attempting to establish an outcome evaluation is the development of a clear statement of objectives by the program staff. It is axiomatic that an outcome evaluation cannot proceed unless adequate objectives have been developed. There are three areas of focus that an objective should address:

- Desired behaviors (for example, a decrease in unprotected sex)
- Specific circumstances (for example, after three hours of intervention)
- Level of performance (for example, decrease sustained at sixty-day follow-up)

Objectives are best derived as part of an interactive process that includes staff and evaluators.

EVALUATION DESIGN

The evaluation design is the overall plan that determines when and from whom measurements will be taken (Fitz-Gibbon and Morris, 1987). A comprehensive design provides both the broad parameters of the evaluation as well as suggests the methodologies and instruments to be used.

It is important to stress that the program administrator should think about the evaluation design *before* program implementation. It is difficult—if not impossible—to go back and change the design after the fact. The evaluation design should be clearly worked out and articulated during program planning stages or, when relevant, reflected in a grant application.

Designs can be of varying degrees of complexity and sophistication. The National Research Council discusses three general evaluation designs: (1) randomized experiments, (2) quasi-experiments, and (3) nonexperimental methods.

Randomized experiments and even quasi-experimental design are usually too sophisticated for most small-scale program evaluations. They are expensive and require substantial expertise. But program managers should not despair if they cannot reach the ideal of randomized experiments. Conducting randomized evaluation is rare in any field. In one nationwide sample of bilingual education programs, for example, evaluations revealed that not one attempted to use a true, randomized control group, and only 36 percent tried to locate a nonrandomized control group for comparison. Moore and Forst (1993) made similar findings in their study of AIDS education and prevention programs in California. No local program in the study used experimental or quasi-experimental methods to test the effectiveness of their interventions.

In quasi-experimental designs, the control group is selected by matching nonparticipants with participants in the program on the basis of specified characteristics. But, for a variety of reasons, even quasi-experimental and matched-control designs are difficult for local program evaluations. First, it is often difficult to acquire "comparable" groups. Programs frequently work with small target populations; there simply are not enough subjects in the target group to form a valid comparison group. Ethical dilemmas also surface. Many AIDS educators are reluctant to deny life-saving information to one group (a control or comparison group) simply for the sake of an experiment. The National Research Council "recognizes that community and political opposition to randomization or to zero treatments may be strong and that enlisting participation in such experiments may be difficult" (National Academy of Sciences, 1991).

Most local program evaluations use nonexperimental methods. A common form of nonexperimental design is the pre–post (also called before-and-after) study. In this design, measurements taken before the intervention are compared with equivalent post-intervention measures to determine changes in the outcome variables that the program was supposed to bring about. The nonexperimental methods usually fall into two types: (1) pre–post testing or (2) post-test only design.

The pre–post method is preferable among the nonexperimental methods. The CDC's guidelines for evaluation of education and prevention programs suggest the use of a "baseline" preprogram measure as a basis for estimating change that occurs as a consequence of these projects. But some programs use the post-test only design. Each has advantages and disadvantages which relate to both theoretical and practical concerns.

One might argue that the main issue in an AIDS education and prevention program is for the target population to attain some level of knowledge, attitude, or behavior regarding HIV infection. It is not necessarily important, from a practical standpoint, whether the clients attained the desired level from the program per se, or whether the clients already had some level of attainment. If one accepts this line of reasoning, it would be justifiable to use a post-test only design. That is, you could give the test following the intervention and determine if the clients have in fact attained the desired levels of knowledge, attitude, or behavior.

It might also be argued that the idea of the program is to *change* the knowledge, attitude, or behavior of the target population. This implies that the program personnel know the levels of knowledge, attitudes, or behavior both before and after the intervention. The pre–post design is thus required. This design will help determine whether the clients had already attained the levels measured before the intervention. This is important, in the long run, because of cost concerns. It is not the most effective utilization of resources to provide interventions if the clients already have the requisite levels of knowledge.

There are also practical considerations in choosing the evaluation design. For many target groups, if not most, time is a scarce commodity. For health educators who have their clients' attention for short periods of time—an hour or less—dispensing what is viewed to be lifesaving information is given the highest priority. Many health educators do not feel they have the luxury of doing both pre- and post-testing. As a consequence, health educators choose only minimal evaluative measurement; the minimal measurement is typically some sort of short post-intervention testing.

Another consideration relates to the large workload that often burdens program staff. Most staff members feel they must concentrate on arranging and providing educational interventions. Spending more effort on evaluation would, in the minds of many staff members, detract from their primary mission—providing critical education to people believed to be desperately in need of it.

These practical considerations are compelling reasons for most program staff members to use post-testing only as their evaluation design. However, a post-test evaluation design will not address many crucial issues. Without using a pre–post evaluation design, program staff cannot determine what and how much different target groups know before the intervention is provided. Without knowing preexisting knowledge levels, health educators cannot assess how to tailor the interventions or presentations to fit the needs of the target population.

More important, not knowing preexisting knowledge levels of clients prevents program staff from determining whether the interventions are superfluous—that is, whether the program is presenting information the target audience already possesses. From a public-policy planning perspective, it is crucial to make rational choices in the allocation of scarce public funds. It is not cost effective to spend money to educate groups of people who already have the requisite knowledge levels. It would be more prudent, and eventually have a greater preventive value, to concentrate resources on those groups who most need the educational interventions. Such resources cannot be so allocated without first determining the specific current knowledge levels of various target populations.

One point must be reiterated. Programs rarely include a theoretical framework to guide their interventions or the outcome measures of those interventions. There are a variety of theoretical orientations or models of health education. One thing all models have in common is their attempt to link knowledge, attitudes, and behavior change. Generally speaking, however, local programs focus only on cognitive knowledge. Program managers should thus try to adopt a theoretical framework for their program and link the goals, objectives, and outcome measures of the evaluation to that theoretical framework.

SAMPLING

From the authors' experience in California, most local AIDS education and prevention programs are relatively small in scale. As a practical matter, such programs can and should use all clients in the evaluation. Sampling is necessary when you are attempting to make generalized statements about a large group—one so big that it would be impossible to reach all of its members. For example, when polling firms release results of public-opinion polls, those polls represent the opinions of a scientifically derived sample of the "public." Whether the survey results reflect actual opinions of the group depends largely on how representative the sample was. However, since selecting a sample is expensive and requires a particular type of expertise, it is our opinion that sampling is probably both unnecessary and overly cumbersome for most programs.

Sampling is a rather technical enterprise, requiring expertise in research methodology. If you need to do sampling for your program evaluation, we recommend that you hire a consultant. (See the subsequent section on consultants.)

PROGRAM DOCUMENTATION:
IT IS OK TO COUNT BEANS

It is a good idea to count and document everything during your program's implementation and ongoing operation. The National Research Council has a formal name for this activity; they call it "standardized administrative reporting." Some people disparagingly call this "bean counting." But, in our opinion, bean counting is a legitimate and worthwhile activity.

There are many things to count and document in education and prevention programs. These include, for example, the characteristics of services delivered (type, to whom, how often), the nature of quality controls for the delivery of services, numbers of voluntary and paid staff, staff qualifications, staff turnover, how many brochures were handed out, and how many times a video was shown. These are just a few of the scores of activities that can be documented.

Some of this documentation may seem mundane. But the resulting data can provide a wealth of information. Thus, according to the National Academy, "the information gathered by an administrative form . . . could provide a reasonably accurate, up-to-date, and comprehensive description of the services being provided by CBOs" (National Academy of Sciences, 1991).

For the most part, program record-keeping systems can be simple and straightforward. This is particularly true for formal educational programs. Most programs should have some sort of log sheet, so that the health educator giving the presentation can count the number in attendance. These attendance sheets can be simply tallied (weekly, monthly, or quarterly) to determine if program objectives are being met. On occasion, programs should have more detailed log sheets, which include some demographic data on attendees. For example, the health educator might note how many and what percentage of the attendees are male or female, from what ethnic groups, and so forth. Such data may be needed, for instance, if the program objectives specify that a particular percentage of the clients be members of an ethnic minority group.

Some record-keeping problems bring into question whether, in some instances, measurable objectives are achieved. The biggest and most persistent problem facing programs is keeping track of clients who had already been contacted through various street outreach methods. Outreach workers normally keep a daily or weekly activity book. The outreach worker is to note each separate contact with a client. However, two specific problems can arise with this method.

First, it is often unclear whether the person contacted by the outreach worker is, in fact, a member of the designated target population. If an IDU outreach worker, for example, gives an educational presentation to a small group of people located in an area where drugs are known to be sold, it is not always possible to determine if all group members are IDUs. Thus, people receiving an educational presentation may be counted as members of a specified target group when that fact has not been established.

A second problem has to do with multiple counting of outreach clients. If a program states in its scope of work that some specified number of clients will be reached, that presumably means a specified number of *different* clients. This is not to suggest that individual clients should not be reached numerous times. Rather, when determining whether the minimum objectives have been met, contract terms intend that clients should be counted separately—that is, unduplicated counts. This, unfortunately, is not always done. Some outreach workers log the number of daily contacts, but not the number of separate contacts. The problem can be exacerbated when there are multiple outreach workers in the same area, sometimes reaching the same clients.

The point is that administrative record keeping (i.e., bean counting) can be problematic; the methodological and logistic issues raised should be addressed before program implementation. Naturally, all contingencies cannot be anticipated in advance; experience frequently brings new problems to light. But, to the extent possible, the program manager should have a standardized administrative record-keeping system in place as soon as possible.

EVALUATION OUTCOMES (MEASURES)

The National Research Council suggests that AIDS education and prevention programs should use any one of three types of outcome measures: (1) biological, (2) behavioral, and (3) psychological.

Biological outcomes typically relate to changes in HIV seroconversion rates. However, such outcome measures are unrealistic for smaller-scale program evaluations. Changes in seroconversion rates, or other biological measures like changes in various STD rates, are long-term measures. While they may be monitored by programs, they should not be selected, at least for small-scale programs, as the primary outcome measures.

Behavioral outcomes, as the name suggests, focus on specific behaviors that the subjects are supposed to change. Behavioral changes can be broken down into "risk-reduction behaviors" and "protective behaviors." Risk-reduction behaviors generally are behaviors that a person avoids doing—that is, it is avoidance behavior. Specifically included are abstinence behaviors, such as not engaging in injection drug use or not engaging in sexual intercourse. Protective behaviors, by contrast, are those in which clients continue to engage in risky acts, but take protective measures, such as using a condom or cleaning a needle with bleach before injection.

Changes in risk behavior will presumably reduce HIV transmission in target populations with high seroprevalence rates and, at the same time, will protect populations in which HIV is not yet well established. Accurate measurements of changes in risk behaviors could be the most relevant indicators of program success. This is why the National Research Council concludes, "behavioral measures should be the primary outcome variables for most AIDS intervention programs" (National Academy of Sciences, 1991).

While behavioral measures are obviously desirable, they present numerous difficulties for smaller-scale programs. First, such measures normally imply that a person will be seen on more than one occasion—that is, followed over time. This is often a mistaken assumption regarding many education and prevention programs, particularly those that target hard-to-reach groups. AIDS education may be a one-shot proposition. However, as programs become more targeted and organized, it will be easier to follow people who engage in high-risk behaviors over time. At that point, behavioral-change outcomes will become more feasible.

Psychological outcome measures appear most appropriate for smaller programs. The National Research Council uses the term "psychological" to designate such variables as knowledge and attitudes. This phraseology is similar to the "knowledge, attitudes, and beliefs" that some states focus on.

Psychological outcomes may simply consist of measures of knowledge acquisition. There are some groups, such as Southeast-Asian refugees, that still have relatively low knowledge levels of HIV transmission and prevention. Continued emphasis on knowledge acquisition is important because, as the National Academy points out, "differences in the degree to which individuals are aware of AIDS, understand which behaviors transmit HIV, and disparage or devalue those who are ill or infected may be important determinants of whether they adopt risk reduction or protective behaviors" (National Academy of Sciences, 1991).

Psychological outcome measures are easier and cheaper for the average program to employ. Thus, "psychological outcomes that involve awareness of AIDS and HIV, knowledge about AIDS and HIV transmission, and attitudes toward those who are infected and ill may be the easiest outcomes to measure and study, in the sense that these measures are easily incorporated in a survey questionnaire" (National Academy of Sciences, 1991).

CHOOSING EVALUATION TOOLS (INSTRUMENTS)

It is one thing to understand the importance of measuring knowledge, attitude, belief, and behavior change; it is another thing to know how to do it. There is more to measurement than meets the eye. That is why, as a practical matter, most programs do not adequately assess these variables.

Program administrators and evaluators face numerous practical and methodological issues. One issue is whether to choose an existing instrument or to devise one specifically for the program at hand. Our general recommendation is that it is better to use existing, validated instruments. However, this rule is true for more standard target groups in the general population. Standardized instruments may not be appropriate for many specific target populations. In this case, it may be necessary to devise your own instrument. This choice, though, is less than ideal, and raises methodological concerns. For example, if the instrument has not been validated, it is unclear whether it is measuring what it is supposed to measure.

There are also cost implications of the measures used. A thorough evaluation will cost a lot of money, relatively speaking. Assessing behavior change in particular would most likely entail following a cohort of clients over time. Such longitudinal studies are difficult to conduct—they are technically more complex and require the commitment of substantial amounts of time and money.

One of the more pressing issues for program staff is making the content and wording of the instruments (tests) appropriate to the reading (literacy) levels of the target population. In many instances, program staff become aware that words used in tests for the general population cannot be understood readily by some hard-to-reach populations. In such instances, we recommend that program staff consult peer educators and find a "street word" that carries the same meaning.

A related problem is devising tests appropriate to non–English-speaking clients. A common procedure is for program staff to translate a version of the test that has been given to similar English-speaking target populations. How the translations are carried out can differ. For example, an in-house, bilingual educator can make the translation. More elaborate procedures can also be used (e.g., hiring a professional translator or having the translation reviewed by a local task force to increase the probability that the questions are appropriately worded).

Some instruments minimize words. California State University at Long Beach psychologists created a test using pictures to be administered to populations with low literacy levels. Methods of HIV transmission were depicted, and participants were asked to indicate those methods which were likely to transmit HIV and those that were not. Approaches to protect oneself from infection (condom use and cleaning needles) were also demonstrated in this approach.

THE FEEDBACK LOOP

As we said before, it is advisable to use the information acquired during the evaluation to monitor how your program is doing—to keep improving the effectiveness of the program. Thus, "process evaluation can also play a role in improving interventions by providing the information necessary to change delivery strategies or program objectives in a changing epidemic" (National Academy of Sciences, 1991).

We are talking about the utilization of evaluation data. Evaluation findings have both instrumental and conceptual uses. Data can be used to make immediate program alterations—called instrumental use. Program evaluation can also change the way managers think about the program—called conceptual use. This distinction could be relevant long after the evaluation is completed. Program administrators must learn to see that they can make decisions that affect their program both in the short term and the long term.

Unfortunately, most program managers do not use evaluation data to improve their programs. In a recent California study, only one program (at a university) conducted a thorough analysis of how well the target populations scored on the questions in the post-test and used that analysis to alter program interventions (Moore and Forst, 1993). Revisions of the educational protocols were not made in the other programs.

This is unfortunate, because using internal evaluation data to improve a program can be relatively easy. For example, it is necessary, but not sufficient, to simply determine the percentage of answers the clients got correct, even though this may be part of your measurable objectives. But you should do more. To improve the program, it is necessary to examine the response patterns to the questions. You may discover that a large percentage of your clients incorrectly answer a question about mosquitos causing AIDS. If so, it is imperative that the health educator spend extra time on this point in the future. Perhaps there is something about that topic or concept that is confusing to the client population. The health educator should alter the presentation to ensure that the clients gain adequate understanding.

There has been a lot of research on the utilization of evaluation. Much research points to the importance of the "personal factor." Managers tend to be busy people who spend relatively little time on a lot of different problems. To have an impact, evaluation results should be communicated in short, easy-to-digest form, preferably orally, rather than in a large technical report. They also should be communicated to those who care about the information. Thus, to improve utilization it is important to find the strategically located persons and address the issues of concern to them.

LOCAL POLITICS AND UTILIZATION

Programs are continuously changing. They have supporters and detractors. Opposition to a program by those who disagree with it will continue no matter what an evaluation shows. Programs serve symbolic and political as well as substantive ends. Programs are often not changed for technical or analytical reasons, but for ideological or political reasons. And there is no such thing as an evaluation that does not have political considerations. Evaluations thus have political as well as program implications. Some people believe that the Reagan administration used cost–benefit analysis as window dressings for its real purpose of deregulating and overturning regulations of the Occupational Safety and Health Administration.

It is important to be aware of these political issues from program design through dissemination of results. The political factors may actually help the program conduct a more thorough evaluation. "If political pressures or heat of controversy make it important that you produce credible information about program efforts, few things will support you better than a well chosen evaluation design" (Fitz-Gibbon and Morris, 1987).

Evaluations are inevitably political in several ways. Evaluations make judgments about programs and therefore become a part of the politics surrounding them. Evaluations are political, no matter how objective or neutral evaluators think they are, because they serve the interests of persons involved in the policy process. If the evaluation finds, for example, that AIDS negotiation-skills classes change behavior for the better, then the evaluation is saying implicitly, if not explicitly, that future policy actions should be influenced by this information. The evaluation is entering the world of political debate.

How should evaluators and administrators respond to the inherently political nature of evaluation? Evaluators should recognize that they cannot always be "objective." At the same time, they should avoid becoming the tools of one particular interest. They can do this by making sure that an array of interested parties are included in the design, implementation, and analysis of the evaluation. In addition, they can attempt to represent interests that are not or cannot be involved (such as those of the clients or targets of the program or the general public). Evaluators and policy analysts should also recognize that evaluations are limited in what they can do. They are but one element of the policy process, and by no means the most important.

WORKING WITH CONSULTANTS

A consultant is a dirty word in some circles. There may be some justification for this tarnished reputation, but consultants can be of great value. They can save the program administrator a lot of time and money. Most importantly, they can help ensure that the program evaluation is successful and effective.

If you have a big program, one with a large budget, we recommend that you hire a consultant (or consulting firm) to conduct the evaluation. It is worth it. It is cost effective in the long run to spend a little extra money for a good evaluation.

For smaller programs, limited budgets will not permit hiring outside experts to conduct an entire evaluation. But it is important to realize that you can hire a consultant on a part-time basis—hourly or daily. Many issues can be resolved in a short period of time. It is particularly desirable to use consulting services at the beginning of the program to ensure a sound design and methodology. Consultants are also useful for addressing particularly technical issues, such as sampling.

Hiring a consultant (or a consulting firm) to conduct the evaluation has other advantages. For one, there is more free time for program staff to do other program work. Moreover, an independent evaluation by a reputable consultant will lend the results of the evaluation enhanced credibility. Colleges and universities are also a possible source of evaluation assistance. Knowledgeable graduate students are often willing to work collaboratively with community-based program staff (on a pro bono basis) to design and implement a program evaluation.

The two-culture theory holds that evaluators and administrators live in different worlds that sometimes have conflicting goals. Evaluators hope to find the facts and generalize about a program. Administrators, by contrast, are interested in specific information about populations in certain situations. These different world views can lead to conflict and dissention. But it does not have to be that way. If you decide to hire a consultant, communicate. Tell the consultant what you want and come to an agreement. Then monitor the consultant's progress.

We include in our definition of consultants what are sometimes called resource specialists. There are many good videos and brochures, for example, and resource consultants know what is available and what is most appropriate for your target population. For example, the CDC-sponsored National AIDS Clearinghouse (1-800-458-5231) or, in California, ETR Associates of Santa Cruz (1-800-321-4407) have full listings of available resources.

You can also improve your internal evaluations with consulting materials already published. For example, you can buy a series of books on program evaluation, published by Sage Publications, that are written by professional evaluators from the UCLA Center for the Study of Evaluation. They also put out a Program Evaluation Kit.

CONCLUSION

Evaluation will likely become an increasingly important component of the program manager's job. As long as citizens, elected officials, and administrators ask questions about the effectiveness of government programs, program evaluation will remain crucial to administration. More and more, evaluation design and methodology are becoming important factors in the granting of funds by government agencies.

It is essential, as a program administrator, to be involved in the evaluation phase of the program from the outset. It is common for an evaluation component to be part of the grant application, so you should be thinking about the evaluation from the time the grant application is being written.

Evaluations are conducted for a variety of reasons, but, ultimately, the main purpose is to provide information for decision making. "Given the seriousness of the disease and the benefits associated with prevention, commitment of adequate resources for careful evaluations of the effectiveness of AIDS prevention programs should be viewed as a wise investment in the future" (National Academy of Sciences, 1991).

Finally, as we said earlier, evaluation of education and prevention programs is not easy, but it is critical. Are we giving the citizens of this country, as well as the clients of our service programs, the best possible health-protecting information and programs? To say, "we don't know" is simply not good enough. The lessons to be learned from good evaluations are far from trivial. Since effective education and prevention programs are valuable, the urgency of doing this difficult work better is, we hope, obvious.

REFERENCES

Fitz-Gibbon, C. T., and L. L. Morris. (1987). *How to Design Program Evaluation*. Newbury Park, Calif.: Sage.

Moore, M. K., and M. L. Forst. (1993). Evaluation of Four San Francisco–Based AIDS Education Programs. Technical report for the San Francisco Department of Public Health, San Francisco, Calif., pp. 3–5.

National Academy of Sciences, National Research Council. (1991). *Evaluating AIDS Prevention Programs*. Washington, D.C.: National Academy of Sciences.

][───────────────

Selected Bibliography

American Association of University Women Educational Foundation. (1991). *Shortchanging Girls. Shortchanging America.* Washington, D.C.: American Association of University Women Educational Foundation.

Bethel, E. Rauh, ed. (1995). *AIDS: Readings on a Global Crisis.* Needham Heights, Mass: Allyn and Bacon.

Blum, H. L. (1981). *Planning for Health.* New York: Human Services Press.

Bogart, K., and N. Stein. (1987). Breaking the Silence: Sexual Harassment in Education. *Peabody Journal of Education* 64(4): 146–163.

Brooks-Gunn, J. (1992). The Impact of Puberty and Sexual Activity upon the Health and Education of Adolescent Girls and Boys. In *Sex Equity and Sexuality in Education,* edited by S. Klein, 97–126. New York: State University of New York Press.

Burkhart, D. (1991). Who Said the Sexual Revolution Is Over? *Medical Aspects of Human Sexuality* 25: 9.

Carnegie Council on Adolescent Development. (1989). *Turning Points: Preparing Youth for the 21st Century.* New York: Carnegie Corporation.

Centers for Disease Control (CDC). (1988a). Guidelines for Effective School Health Education to Prevent the Spread of AIDS. *Morbidity and Mortality Weekly Report* 37 (January 29 supplement): 1–14.

Centers for Disease Control (CDC). (1988b). HIV-Related Beliefs, Knowledge, and Behaviors among High School Students. *Morbidity and Mortality Weekly Report* 37: 717–721.

Centers for Disease Control (CDC). (1988c). Prevalence of Human Immunodeficiency Virus Antibody in U.S. Active-Duty Military Personnel. *Morbidity and Mortality Weekly Report* 37: 461–463.

Centers for Disease Control (CDC). (1989a). *Annual Report.* Atlanta: CDC, Division of STD/HIV Prevention.

Centers for Disease Control (CDC). (1989b). Update: Heterosexual Transmission of Acquired Immunodeficiency Syndrome and Human Immunodeficiency Virus Infection—United States. *Morbidity and Mortality Weekly Report* 38: 423–433.

Centers for Disease Control (CDC). (1990a). HIV/AIDS Surveillance Report: August. Atlanta: CDC.

Centers for Disease Control (CDC). (1990b). HIV/AIDS Surveillance: June. Atlanta: CDC.

Centers for Disease Control (CDC). (1991a). *Division of STD/HIV Prevention Annual Report, 1990.* Atlanta: CDC.

Centers for Disease Control (CDC). (1991b). Publicly Funded HIV Counseling and Testing, United States, 1990. *Morbidity and Mortality Weekly Report* 40: 666–669.

Centers for Disease Control (CDC). (1992). HIV/AIDS Surveillance: October. Atlanta: CDC.

Centers for Disease Control (CDC). (1993). HIV/AIDS Surveillance, Second Quarter Edition.

Centers for Disease Control (CDC). (1994). HIV Infection Cases by Sex, Age and Diagnosis and Race/Ethnicity. *HIV/AIDS Surveillance Report* 6(2): 34.

Centers for Disease Control (CDC). (1995). HIV/AIDS Surveillance Summary as of May 1, 1995. Atlanta: CDC.

Chris, Cynthia. (1990). Transmission Issues for Women. In *Women, AIDS, & Activism,* edited by Cynthia Chris and Monica Pearl, 17–25. Boston: South End Press.

Cohen, Judith B. (1993). HIV Risk among Women Who Have Sex with Women. *San Francisco Epidemiologic Bulletin* 9(4): 25–29.

Communication Technologies. (1993). *A Call of a New Generation of AIDS Prevention for Gay and Bisexual Men in San Francisco.* San Francisco: Communication Technologies.

Cranston, K. (1992). HIV Education for Gay, Lesbian, and Bisexual Youth: Personal Risk, Personal Power, and the Community of Conscience. In *Coming Out of the Classroom Closet,* edited by Karen M. Harbeck. New York: Harrington Park Press.

DiClemente, R. L. (1992). Epidemiology of AIDS, HIV Prevalence, and HIV Incidence among Adolescents. *Journal of School Health* 62(7): 325–330.

Dorney, J. (forthcoming). Educating toward Resistance: A Task for Women Teaching Girls. *Youth and Society.*

Ephraim, J. C. (1992). "Developing an STD and HIV/AIDS Program for the Incarcerated Population." Workshop excerpts from the National Skills Building Conference.

Erikson, E. (1968). *Identity, Youth and Crisis.* New York: W. W. Norton.

Fine, M. (1993). Sexuality, Schooling and Adolescent Females: The Missing Discourse of Desire. In *Beyond Silenced Voices: Class, Race and Gender in United States Schools,* edited by L. Weiss and M. Fine, 77–99. New York: State University of New York Press.

Fitz-Gibbon, C. T., and L. L. Morris. (1987). *How to Design Program Evaluation.* Newbury Park, Calif.: Sage.

Freire, P. (1970). *Pedagogy of the Oppressed.* New York: Seabury Press.

Freire, Paulo. (1973). *Education and Conscientizacao* (Education for Critical Consciousness). New York: Seabury Press.

Freire, Paulo. (1976). Pedagogy of the Oppressed (summary). In *The Planning of Change*, edited by W. G. Bennis et al. 3d ed. New York: Holt, Rinehart & Winston.

Fullilove, M. (1991). Testimony before the National Commission on AIDS: Adolescents and HIV Disease. 13 March, Chicago.

Gilligan, C., N. Lyons, and T. Hanmer. (1990). *Making Connections: The Relational Worlds of Adolescent Girls at Emma Willard School*. Cambridge: Harvard University Press.

Gold, R. (1992). Situational Factors and Thought Processes Associated with Unprotected Intercourse in Young Gay Men. *AIDS* 6: 1021–1030.

Green, L., and M. Kreuter. (1991). *Health Promotion Planning: An Educational and Environmental Approach*. Mountain View, Calif.: Mayfield.

Greenspan, J. (1991). AIDS in Prison: The National Perspective. *California AIDS Clearinghouse Reviewer* 3(1): 4.

Gross, J. (1993). "Second Wave of AIDS Feared by Officials in San Francisco." *The New York Times*, 11 December, pp. 1, 8.

Hammett, T. M., L. Harrold, M. Gross, and J. Epstein. (1994). 1992 Update: HIV/AIDS in Correctional Facilities. Washington, D.C.: U.S. Department of Justice, National Institute of Justice, pp. 14–18.

Hays, R. B., S. M. Kegeles, and T. J. Coates. (1990). High Risk Taking among Young Gay Men. *AIDS* 4: 901–907.

Healthy Boston Coalition Survey. (1995). Forthcoming.

Hernández, Eberardo S. (1978). *Plan de Cinco Años*. Oakland, Calif.: La Clínica De La Raza.

Hernández, Eberardo S. (1983). *Considerations For Community Organizers*. Oakland, Calif.: La Clínica De La Raza.

Hessol, N. A., G. W. Rutherford, A. R. Lifson, et al. (1988). "The Natural History of HIV Infection in a Cohort of Homosexual and Bisexual Men: A Decade of Follow-Up." Proceedings of the Fourth International Conference on AIDS, Stockholm, Sweden, abstract 4096.

Heyward, W. L., and J. W. Curran. (1988). The Epidemiology of AIDS in the U.S. *Scientific American* 259(4): 72–81.

Hoover, D. R., A. Munoz, V. Carey, et al. (1991). Estimating the 1978–1990 and Future Spread of Human Immunodeficiency Virus Type 1 in Subgroups of Homosexual Men. *American Journal of Epidemiology* 134: 1190–1205.

Hope, Ann, and Sally Timmel. (1984). *Training for Transformation*. Gweru, Zimbabwe: Mambo Press.

Howard, M. (1993). Testimony before the National Commission on AIDS: Prevention Strategies in the Workplace and Schools: Current Challenges. 11 March, Austin, Texas.

Humes, S., and M. Waters. (1992). A Process Evaluation of "Eroticizing Safer Sex." New York: Gay Men's Health Crisis.

Joseph, J., S. Montgomer, J. Kirscht, R. Kessler, D. Ostrow, D. Emmons, and J. Phair. (1987). Perceived Risk of AIDS: Assessing the Behavioral and Psychosocial Consequences in a Cohort of Gay Men. *Journal of Applied Social Psychology* 17(3): 231–250.

Kaplan, Helen Singer. (1987). *The Real Truth about Women and AIDS: How to Eliminate the Risks without Giving up Love and Sex.* New York: Fireside Books.

Kayal, P. (1993). The Sociological Imagination in AIDS Prevention Education among Gay Men. *The Social and Behavioral Aspects of AIDS. Advances in Medical Sociology* 3: 201–221.

Kilbourne, B. W., J. W. Buehler, and M. F. Rogers. (1990). AIDS as a Cause of Death in Children, Adolescents, and Young Adults. *American Journal of Public Health* 80(4): 499–550.

Kim, H. (1991). Do You Have Eyelashes? In *Women, Girls and Psychotherapy: Reframing Resistance,* edited by C. Gilligan, A. Rogers, and D. Tolman, 201–212. New York: Haworth Press.

Lemp, G., G. Nieri, and the San Francisco Department of Public Health AIDS Office. (1994). Seroprevalence of HIV and Risk Behaviors among Young Homosexual and Bisexual Men: The San Francisco/Berkeley Young Men's Survey. *Journal of the American Medical Association* 272: 449–454.

Leonard, Zoe. (1990). Lesbians in the AIDS Crisis. In *Women, AIDS, & Activism,* edited by Cynthia Chris and Monica Pearl, 113–118. Boston: South End Press.

Levine, M. (1979). *Gay Ghetto.* New York: Harper & Row.

Maguen, S. (1991). Teen Suicide: The Government's Cover-Up and America's Lost Children. *The Advocate,* 24 September.

Martin, J. (1988). Psychological Consequences of AIDS-Related Bereavement among Gay Men. *Journal of Consulting and Clinical Psychology* 56(6): 856–862.

Masters, W., and V. Johnson. (1979). *Homosexuality in Perspective.* New York: Bantam Books.

Mayer, K. (1995). Epidemiology and Biological Factors. Presentation at the Summit on the Reduction of New HIV Infections among Gay Men in Massachusetts, 8–9 June, Boston.

Mayer K., and G. Seage. (1994). HIV Seroprevalence among Gay College Men in Boston. Poster presented at the Tenth International Conference on AIDS, 7–12 August, Yokohama, Japan.

McKenzie, Nancy, ed. (1991). *The AIDS Reader: Social, Political, Ethnical Issues.* New York: Penguin Books.

McKnight, J., and J. Kretzman. (1984). Community Organizing in the 80's: Toward a Post-Alinsky Agenda. *Social Policy* 14: 15–17.

McWhirter, D., and A. Mattison. (1984). *The Male Couple: How Relationships Develop.* Englewood Cliffs, N.J.: Prentice-Hall.

Mikel Brown, L., and C. Gilligan. (1990). The Psychology of Women and the Development of Girls. Paper presented at the annual meeting of the American Educational Research Association.

Miller, H., C. Turner, and L. Moses, eds. (1990). *AIDS: The Second Decade.* Washington, D.C.: National Academy Press.

Miller, J. (1991). The Development of Women's Sense of Self. In *Women's Growth in Connection: Writings from the Stone Center,* edited by J. Jordan, A. Kaplan, J. Miller, I. Stiver, and J. Surrey, 11–26. New York: Guilford Press.

Miller, R., K. Bratholt, R. Frederick, A. Grogan, B. Johnson, J. Kosciw, D. McDonagh, M. Manalansan, and A. Motta Moraes. (1993). *An Evaluation of the "Keep It Up!" Workshop and Support Groups: Final Report.* New York: Gay Men's Health Crisis.

Moore, M. K., and M. L. Forst. (1993). Evaluation of Four San Francisco-Based AIDS Education Programs. Technical report for the San Francisco Department of Public Health, San Francisco, Calif.

Morgan, W. M., and J. W. Curran. (1986). Acquired Immunodeficiency Syndrome: Current and Future Trends. *Public Health Reports* 101: 459–465.

National Academy of Sciences, National Research Council. (1991). *Evaluating AIDS Prevention Programs.* Washington, D.C.: National Academy of Sciences.

Newman, B., and P. Newman. (1987). *Development through Life: A Psychosocial Approach.* Chicago: Dorsey Press.

New York State Department of Health. (April 1994). Criminal Justice Initiative Prison Program. Focus on AIDS in New York State. Albany, N.Y.: New York State Department of Health.

Odets, W. (1990). The Homosexualization of AIDS. *FOCUS: A Guide to AIDS Research and Counseling* 5(11): 1–2.

Odets, W. (1994a). AIDS Education and Harm Reduction for Gay Men: Psychological Approaches to the 21st Century. *AIDS and Public Policy Journal* 9(1): 1–20.

Odets, W. (1994b). Psychosocial and Educational Challenges for the Gay and Bisexual Male Communities. Paper presented at the American Association of Physicians for Human Rights, AIDS Prevention Summit, 15–17 July, Dallas, Texas.

Odets, W. (1995). The Fatal Mistakes of AIDS Education. *San Francisco Bay Times* 15(41): 3–7.

Osborne Association. (1995). "AIDS in Prison Project Fact Sheet." New York: Osborne Association.

Patton, Cindy. (1990). *Inventing AIDS.* New York: Routledge.

Patton, Cindy. (1991). Safe Sex and the Pornographic Vernacular. In *How Do I Look?*, edited by The Bad Object-Choices Collective, 31–63. Seattle: Bay Press.

Patton, Cindy. (1994). *Last Served? Gendering the HIV Pandemic.* Bristol, Pa.: Taylor & Francis.

Paul, J., R. Stall, M. Crosby, et al. (1994). Correlates of Sexual Risk-Taking among Gay Male Substance Abusers. *Addiction* 89: 971–983.

Prieur, A. (1990). Norwegian Gay Men: Reasons for Continued Practice of Unsafe Sex. *AIDS Education and Prevention: An Interdisciplinary Journal* 2(2): 109–115.

Prochaska, J., C. DiClemente, and J. Norcross. (1992). In Search of How People Change: Applications to Addictive Behaviors. *American Psychologist* 47(9): 1102–1113.

Reed, D. (1981). Social Education. In *Education for Building a People's Movement.* Boston: South End Press.

Remafedi, G. (1991). Risk Factors for Attempted Suicide in Gay and Bisexual Youth. *Pediatrics* 87: 869–875.

Remafedi, G. (1994). Predictors on Unprotected Intercourse among Gay and Bisexual Youth: Knowledge, Beliefs and Behavior. *Pediatrics* 4: 901–907.

Remick, S., and S. Szebenyi. (1994). The Primary Care of HIV Infection in a Correctional-Facility Setting. *The AIDS Reader* 4(3): 79.

Richardson, Diane. (1994). Inclusions and Exclusions: Lesbians, HIV and AIDS. In *AIDS: Setting a Feminist Agenda*, edited by Lesley Doyal, Jennie Naidoo, and Tamsin Wilton, 159–170. Bristol, Pa.: Taylor & Francis.

Robinson, T., and J. Ward. (1991). A Belief in Self Far Greater than Anyone's Disbelief: Cultivating Resistance among African American Female Adolescents. In *Women, Girls and Psychotherapy: Reframing Resistance*, edited by C. Gilligan, A. Rogers, and D. Tolman. New York: Haworth Press.

Rosenburg, P. S., R. J. Biggar, and J. J. Goedert. (1994). Declining Age at HIV Infection in the United States. *New England Journal of Medicine* 330: 789–790.

Sadker, M., and D. Sadker. (1994). *Failing at Fairness: How America's Schools Cheat Girls.* New York: Charles Scribner's Sons.

Sadownick, D. (1994). Untamed Youth. *Genre* (March): 37–43, 92.

San Francisco Department of Public Health, Prevention Services Branch, AIDS Office. (1993). Health Behaviors among Lesbians and Bisexual Women: A Community-Based Women's Health Survey. San Francisco: Department of Public Health.

San Francisco Department of Public Health, Surveillance Branch, AIDS Office. (1993). HIV Seroprevalence and Risk Behaviors among Lesbians and Bisexual Women: The 1993 San Francisco/Berkeley Women's Survey. San Francisco: Department of Public Health.

San Francisco Department of Public Health, Surveillance Branch, AIDS Office. (1995a). AIDS Surveillance Report. San Francisco: Department of Public Health.

San Francisco Department of Public Health, Surveillance Branch, AIDS Office. (1995b). HIV Seroprevalance Report. San Francisco: Department of Public Health.

Sapon-Shevin, M., and J. Goodman. (1992). Learning to Be the Opposite Sex: Sexuality Education and Sexual Scripting in Early Adolescence. In *Sexuality and the Curriculum: The Politics and Practices of Sexuality Education*, edited by J. Sears, 89–105. New York: Teachers' College Press.

Schinke, S. P., G. J. Botvin, M. A. Orlandi, R. P. Schilling, and A. N. Gordon. (1990). African-American and Hispanic-American Adolescents, HIV Infection, and Preventive Intervention. *AIDS Education and Prevention* 2(4): 305–312.

Schneider, Beth E., and Nancy E. Stoller. (1994). *Women Resisting AIDS: Feminist Strategies of Empowerment.* Philadelphia: Temple University Press.

Sears, J. (1992). Dilemmas and Possibilities of Sexuality Education: Reproducing the Body Politic. In *Sexuality and the Curriculum: The Politics and Practices of Sexuality Education*, edited by J. Sears, 7–33. New York: Teachers' College Press.

Shernoff, M., and D. J. Bloom. (1991). Designing Effective AIDS Prevention Workshops for Gay and Bisexual Men. *AIDS Education and Prevention* 3(1): 31–46.

Shimmin, Rita, ed. (1995). *HIV Prevention Manual*. Berkeley, Calif.: The National Lesbian/Bisexual Women's HIV Prevention Project and City of Berkeley Health and Human Services.

Silin, J. (1992). School Based HIV/AIDS Education: Is there Safety in Safer Sex? In *Sexuality and the Curriculum: The Politics and Practices of Sexuality Education*, edited by J. Sears, 267–283. New York: Teachers' College Press.

Smart, G. (1995). Barriers to Effective AIDS Education for the Population of Gay Males between the Ages of 15 to 25. Paper presented at the Summit on the Reduction of New HIV Infections among Gay Men in Massachusetts, 8–9 June, Boston.

Smith, B., and C. Dailard. (1994). Female Prisoners and AIDS: On the Margins of Public Health and Social Justice. *AIDS and Public Policy* 9(2): 811.

Solomon, Nancy. (1992). Risky Business. *OUT/LOOK* 4(4): 46–52.

Stall, R. (1994). Intertwining Epidemics? A Short History of Research on the Relationship between Substance Use and the AIDS Epidemic among Gay Men. Paper Presented at the Summit on HIV Prevention for Gay Men, Bisexuals, and Lesbians at Risk, Dallas, Texas.

Stanton, B., M. Black, V. Keane, and S. Feigelman. (1990). HIV Risk Behaviors in Young Black People: Can We Benefit from 30 Years of Research Experience? *AIDS and Public Policy Journal* 5: 17–23.

Stevens, Patricia E. (1993). HIV Risk Reduction for Three Subgroups of Lesbian and Bisexual Women in San Francisco—Year One: Project Evaluation Report. San Francisco: Lyon-Martin Women's Health Services.

Stevens, Patricia E., and Joanne M. Hall. (1994). HIV Risk Reduction for Lesbians and Bisexual Women in San Francisco—Year Two: Year End Evaluation Report. San Francisco: Lyon-Martin Women's Health Services.

Surucam, H. (1994). Study: 20% of Adults Have Gay Impulses. *New York Newsday*, 18 August.

Stine, G. (1993). *Acquired Immune Deficiency Syndrome: Biological, Medical, Social, and Legal Issues*. Englewood Cliffs, N.J.: Prentice-Hall.

Surrey, J. (1991). The Self-in-Relation: A Theory of Women's Development. In *Women's Growth in Connection: Writings from the Stone Center*, edited by J. Jordan, A. Kaplan, J. Miller, I. Stiver, and J. Surrey, 51–66. New York: Guilford Press.

Thomas, Trish. (1994). Dykes Face AIDS. *SF Weekly* 13(23): 12–15.

Tolman, D. (1991). Adolescent Girls, Women and Sexuality: Discerning Dilemmas of Desire. In *Women, Girls, and Psychotherapy: Reframing Resistance*, edited by C. Gilligan, A. Rogers, and D. Tolman, 55–69. New York: Haworth Press.

Tross, S. (1986). Psychological Impact of AIDS Spectrum Disorders in New York City. Presentation at the American Psychological Association Annual Meeting, Washington, D.C.

U.S. Department of Justice. (1993). *Survey of State Prison Inmates, 1991*. Washington, D.C.: Bureau of Justice Statistics.

Van Vugt, Johannes P., ed. (1994). *AIDS Prevention and Services: Community Based Research.* Westport, Conn.: Bergin and Garvey.

Vlahov, D., F. Brewer, and K. Castro. (1991). Prevalence of Antibody to HIV-1 among Entrants to U.S. Correctional Facilities. *Journal of the American Medical Association* 265: 1129–1132.

Wallerstein, Nina, and Edward Bernstein. (1988). Empowerment Education: Freire's Ideas Adapted to Health Education. *Health Education Quarterly* 15(4): 379–394.

Ward, J., and J. Taylor. (1992). Sexuality Education for Immigrant and Minority Students: Developing a Culturally Appropriate Curriculum. In *Sexuality and the Curriculum: The Politics and Practices of Sexuality Education,* edited by J. Sears, 183–202. New York: Teachers' College Press.

Wendell, D., I. Onorato, D. Allen, E. McCray, and P. Sweeney. (1990). Seroprevalence among Adolescents and Young Adults in Selected Clinic Settings, United States, 1988–90. Paper presented at the Sixth International Conference on AIDS, San Francisco, California.

Werner, David. (1980). Health Care & Human Dignity: A Subjective Look at Community-Based Rural Health Programs in Latin America. *Contact,* Special Series, 3: 91–95.

Werner, David, and Bill Bower. (1982). *Helping Health Workers Learn.* Palo Alto, Calif.: The Hesperian Foundation.

Whatley, M. (1992). Goals for Sex-Equitable Sexuality Education. In *Sex Equity and Sexuality in Education,* edited by S. Klein, 83–95. New York: State University of New York Press.

Index

][————————————————

About the Editors
and Contributors

ROBERT L. BARRET is Professor of Counselor Education at the University of North Carolina at Charlotte, and a psychologist in private practice. He is a member of the senior faculty for the American Psychological Association's Project HOPE, a federally funded project that trains psychologists to train other psychologists to provide mental-health services to persons with HIV disease. He is the coauthor of *Gay Fathers* and a gay activist in North Carolina.

MARY BENTLEY is associate professor in the Department of Health Promotion and Human Movement at Ithaca College in Ithaca, New York. She received her Doctorate in Health Education from the University of Maryland in 1990. She is the founder and creator of the Abiquiu Series on Women, and has been a health education teacher in both middle and high schools.

BRIAN T. BYRNES currently is the manager of gay male education at AIDS Action Committee in Boston, Massachusetts. With an academic background in the humanities, Mr. Byrnes entered into AIDS education and prevention work as a sexuality educator for the Planned Parenthood League of Massachusetts. Since then, he was the AIDS Public Information Coordinator and then the Assistant Director of AIDS Education and Prevention for the Massachusetts Department of Public Health.

ELIZABETH R. COCINA is the Manager of Education and Training in the Community Education Program of the Houston Area Women's Center. She supervises the training for the agency, including all publications, volunteer training, and professional inservices.

JAMES F. DUFFIELD received a bachelor of arts degree from St. Francis College, Brooklyn, New York, and a Master of Social Welfare from the Columbia University School of Social Work. From 1989 to the present, he has been the Director of Training for the City of New York, Division of AIDS Services. He specializes in HIV/AIDS education and training for criminal justice populations.

MARTIN L. FORST is a social scientist specializing in health-care evaluation at the URSA Institute in San Francisco. He received his bachelor's degree in psychology at the University of California at Berkeley. He also has a master's and doctorate degree in criminology from the University of California at Berkeley. He has worked on numerous research projects in the field of health education, specializing in HIV/AIDS education since 1985.

KATHRYN HERR is an assistant professor in the College of Education at the University of New Mexico; she teaches for the Divisions of Teacher Preparation and Language, Literacy, and Sociocultural Studies. Current research interests include the fit or lack of fit between school structures and curriculum and diverse students.

JAMES M. HOLMES is an adjunct lecturer at the Hunter College School of Health Sciences. Formerly, he was coordinator of training at Gay Men's Health Crisis, and is a psychotherapist in private practice in New York City.

STEVEN HUMES worked in a variety of positions at Gay Men's Health Crisis, culminating in his appointment as Director of AIDS Prevention in 1993. Since leaving the Gay Men's Health Crisis in 1994, he has served as Library Services Coordinator at the National Hemophilia Foundation. Mr. Humes was also the AIDS Program Coordinator at the American Red Cross in Greater New York and cofounded and led the AIDS Task Force of Winston–Salem, North Carolina, in the mid-1980s. He holds a master's degree in vocal performance from the Cleveland Institute of Music.

MARY K. IRVINE works in the public-health field as a research associate at Polaris Research and Development, Inc. of San Francisco, California. She graduated Phi Beta Kappa with a bachelor of arts degree in women's studies from Wesleyan University. While completing college, she served as a speakers' bureau panelist, facilitated workshops for incoming students on issues of sexuality and coming out, and worked with direct action groups like East Bay Queer Nation. Through Polaris, she is currently doing support work for the San Francisco HIV prevention planning effort. Mary is a lesbian-turned-bisexual, youth-turning adult.

MICHAEL JANG is the President of Four Winds Research of San Francisco, California. Mr. Jang was responsible for the implementation of the first statewide evaluation of AIDS education and prevention programs for the State of California Office of AIDS, Department of Health Services. He has since specialized in the evaluation of HIV/AIDS education programs for Asian and Pacific Islander populations. Mr. Jang holds a bachelor of arts and master's degree from the University of California at Berkeley.

MEREDITH LARSON worked as the HIV Prevention Specialist for Larkin Street Youth Services' Drop-in Center from 1993 to 1995. She is currently enrolled in a graduate public-health program at the University of North Carolina at Chapel Hill; she expects to receive her MPH in health behavior and health education in Spring 1997.

LILLIAN LIOEANJIE is a native New Yorker and holds a BA in Sociology and an MPH in health education communication. Her competence working with adolescents was gained in the South Bronx of New York City; Oakland, California; and, recently, as an AIDS education coordinator and case manager for an HIV/AIDS education intervention program targeting blacks in New Orleans, Louisiana.

MELINDA K. MOORE is senior research associate at the URSA Institute in San Francisco, California. She has worked in the field of HIV/AIDS education, prevention, and evaluation for the past ten years. Ms. Moore has evaluated numerous HIV/AIDS education and prevention programs at the national, state, and local levels. She specializes in health education programs targeting women. She holds a Master of Public Administration degree, specializing in public health.

ADAM ROBINSON has an MA in Clinical/Community Psychology from the University of North Carolina, Charlotte, and a BS in Psychology and Fine Arts from Guilford College, Greensboro, NC. He is a cofounder of Time Out Youth, Inc., a support agency for gay, lesbian, bisexual, and questioning youth, and has helped found several campus organizations for sexual-minority youth. Research interests include those issues at the intersection of health and mental health, such as suicide, HIV risk-reduction promotion, and the special needs of minority youth.

CHRIS SANDOVAL is currently the director of the Multicultural AIDS Resource Center of California (MARCC) at Polaris Research and Development, and a fifteen-year pioneer of the AIDS epidemic. His experience runs the gamut from AIDS chaplaincy and hospice worker, to Deputy Director of the Shanti Project (the first HIV care and treatment provider in the nation), to Director of AIDS Services in Santa Clara County, the largest of the nine Bay Area counties. He has an international reputation as an expert in the field of managing diversity and cross-cultural communication. He was principal architect and chair for the first Cultural Issues Track, which premiered at the Seventh National AIDS Update Conference in San Francisco, in 1995.

MELISSA SCHATZ has worked with high-risk children and adolescents for over a decade, particularly in the areas of substance-abuse prevention and HIV prevention. She has a BA in English from San Francisco State University, California, and is currently working toward her Master of Social Work at San Jose State University, California.

CASSANDRA R. THOMAS is the Director of the Rape Crisis Program at the Houston Area Women's Center, where she supervises all sexual-assault program activities, serves as a media spokesperson for sexual-violence issues, and provides expert testimony in sexual-assault cases. Included in her media appearances have been *Prime Time Live, Nightline's* "Men, Sex and Rape," and *20/20's* "Pushed to the Edge." Ms. Thomas is also the immediate past president of the National Coalition Against Sexual Assault.

SUSANA HENNESSEY TOURÉ is a health educator with a master's degree in public health from the University of California at Berkeley. Between 1979 and 1992, she worked with La Clínica De La Raza, a community health center that serves Latinos in Oakland, California. In that capacity, she supervised the Community Health Education program (Casa CHE) and developed and implemented popular health education programs in the community committed to promoting social justice and health. She is currently with the San Francisco Department of Public Health, Tobacco Free Project.

CASSANDRA HERNÁNDEZ VIVES is a health educator with a bachelor of arts degree in health education from San Francisco State University. She worked for many years at La Clínica De La Raza as a health educator with Casa CHE and later became supervisor of that program. She continues at La Clínica and develops and implements community health education projects that integrate popular education ideas from Latin America and address a variety of community concerns to promote social justice.

ISBN 0-275-94904-4

9 0 0 0 0>

EAN

9 780275 949044

HARDCOVER BAR CODE